"It's just been fantastic."
—Warren Tenney
NY Attorney

"On the basis of a flight fr[...]
I followed the Anti-Jet-L[...]
disorientation. Previously.[...]
—Doroth[...]

"…your diet…worked extremely well for me in a recent trip to and from Italy."
—Louis J. Cohn
Chicago Attorney

"…your Anti-Jet-Lag diet…worked well for me and I arrived in Milan ready to go to work."
—Eugene Callen
President, Callen Manufacturing

"It worked wonderfully! The Detroit-London through-the-night-direct-to-all-day-meetings was never so easy. All along the way through Europe and the Middle East I gave out copies of the diet."
—Maurita Peterson Holland
Head, Technology Libraries

"…it worked perfectly. I was able to do a full day's work immediately on arrival in both directions."
—F. Lincoln Vogel
Department of Electrical Engineering
and Science
University of Pennsylvania

"…I have used your Anti-Jet-Lag diet on two occasions in the last couple of months, both times with great success…I have in turn shared it with no less than thirty people."
—J. D. Weathers
Engineer

"My wife and I…were amazed at the excellent results."
—Harry Wassall
Consulting Geologist

"Going on the Anti-Jet-Lag diet is an essential part of preparing for any trip."
—Arlene Friedman
Mach II Travel Agency

"Thank you for your fine contribution to humanity."
—Office of Public Liaison
The White House

"Thank you for your good book; it was well written and sorely needed."
—John D. Lange
Department of the Treasury

"For the vacationer who doesn't want to miss a minute of sight-seeing abroad, for the business executive who must be sharp at a meeting..."
—Jane Brody
New York Times

"The program...worked perfectly."
—*Milwaukee Journal*

"Ehret...has testimony from thousands of military and industrial executives who have used it [the jet lag diet] in the past few years."
—*Washington Post*

"Dr. Charles F. Ehret has found a way to...reduce or eliminate jet lag."
—*Family Weekly*

"Arm yourself with *Overcoming Jet Lag*."
—United Press International

"...a plan that's designed to ease the body into acting the way it should after a long trip by air."
—*New York Daily News*

OVERCOMING
JET LAG

OVERCOMING
JET LAG

By Dr. Charles F. Ehret
and Lynne Waller Scanlon

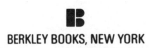

BERKLEY BOOKS, NEW YORK

OVERCOMING JET LAG

A Berkley Book / published by arrangement with
the authors

PRINTING HISTORY
Berkley trade paperback edition / April 1983

The Penguin Putnam Inc. World Wide Web site address is
http://www.penguinputnam.com

ISBN: 0-425-09936-9

BERKLEY®
Berkley Books are published by The Berkley Publishing Group,
a division of Penguin Putnam Inc.,
375 Hudson Street, New York, New York 10014.
BERKLEY and the "B" design
are trademarks belonging to Penguin Putnam Inc.

PRINTED IN THE UNITED STATES OF AMERICA

30   29   28   27   26   25   24   23

DEDICATION
Charles F. Ehret

To Dorothy, through times and time zones distant past and yet to come—*"ensemble, tout semble plus beau."*

DEDICATION
Lynne Waller Scanlon

To my brothers, Mark and Henry, and to their partner, Tom Grill—supportive, generous, good humored, and authors in their own right.

ACKNOWLEDGMENT
Charles F. Ehret

This book reflects the industry and experiences of many people over the course of nearly forty years of work in the young field that we now know as Chronobiology. I am especially grateful to Dr. E. L. Powers of the University of Texas, who first suggested to me, in 1946, that cells may have clocks; to Drs. Van R. Potter, the University of Wisconsin, and Kenneth R. Dobra, the University of Louisville, who collaborated with me in the earliest experiments on the chronobiotic action of the methyl xanthine drugs; to Drs. John J. Wille, the Mayo Clinic, Gregory Antipa, San Francisco State University, and Kenneth R. Groh, Argonne National Laboratory, who worked in my lab at Argonne, showing that food plays a role as a circadian clock synchronizer in free living cells and later in whole animals; and to Drs. Richard Wurtman and John Fernstrom of the Massachusetts Institute of Technology, whose studies on the role of nutrition in determining neurochemical changes in the brain provoked much of the work in many parts of the world that followed up on these early studies.

There are scores of unsung pioneers who, since the earliest days of transmeridional travel, monitored resolutely their physiological and performance rhythms on many long-distance trips. In the forefront of these pioneers are Drs. Franz and Erna Halberg and Dr. Erhard Haus of the University of Minnesota, Dr. L. E. Scheving of the University of Arkansas, and the late Dr. Howard Levine of the New Britain (Connecticut) General Hospital. For their contributions to our best understandings of psychomotor and psychological performance rhythms, we are indebted to Drs. Peter Colquhoun, Simon Folkard, and Timothy Monk, the University of Sussex. For their experimental studies of larger groups of human subjects in transmeridional flight, I owe a lasting debt to Drs. K. E. Klein and H. M. Wegmann of the West German Institute for Aviation Medicine, to Dr. Takashi Sasaki of Kumamoto University, and especially to Major R. Curtis Graeber of the Walter Reed Army Institute of Research.

To the many volunteers and contributors to our own program, and enthusiasts in reporting on its efficacy, I extend my thanks, especially to Henry Cernota and members of the Automotive Transportation Supervisors of Chicago, to Joseph T. Benich and his nomadic Nomads of Detroit, to Robert Phelps of the Boston Globe, to Dr. and Mrs. James Sim of St. Catherines, Ontario, to Warren S. Tenney of New York City, and to Betty and John Menke of Scarsdale, New York. These people were in the vanguard of an increasingly appreciative and demanding public who made perfectly clear to me the need for such a book as this.

This book would never have come to fruition without the professional skill and perseverance of my talented co-author, Lynne Waller Scanlon of New York City. It was she who guided the project through proposal development, placement of the book, and, most important, translation of the esoteric terms and jargon of contemporary biological science into readable and comprehensible form for the general reader.

Special thanks go to my wife, Dorothy Armstrong Ehret, for her indefatigable secretarial help, excellent editorial assistance, and continuous encouragement through all phases of the project.

ACKNOWLEDGMENT
Lynne Waller Scanlon

I would like to thank Charles Ehret, my esteemed co-author, for his unflagging support of a project that weathered the folding of a major publishing house, the dissociation of agent and authors, and the negotiating of multiple contract offers.

I would also like to extend thanks to Linda Healey, our fine editor at Berkley Publishing, and to Nancy Crawford, who had the original idea for this book.

TABLE OF CONTENTS

CHAPTER ONE

THE TRAVELER'S #1 COMPLAINT: JET LAG

In 1963, Lowell Thomas, the famous radio and film commentator who made the very first broadcasts from an airplane and from a ship, and whose sonorous baritone reached billions during his forty-five-year career, was hospitalized because of muscular tremors, extreme fatigue, fainting and vertigo. The physicians attending Lowell suspected that he had had a heart attack, but the diagnosis could not be confirmed through traditional medical methods. Suddenly, the crux of the problem dawned on Lowell; he realized that he had been continually crisscrossing the globe for months in pursuit of news stories. In fact, he felt he had probably crossed all twenty-four time zones at least twice. Indeed, his acute symptoms were merely masquerading as those of a heart attack. In reality, he was experiencing severe jet lag.

****

Greg Luganis, a 1979 finalist on the United States Olympic Diving Team, reported on NBC's "Sports Year '79—A Salute to the Champions" that the reason he had struck his head on the ten-meter platform during a reverse dive at the Olympic trials in Moscow in 1979, was that his acrobatic skills and precision timing had been dramatically affected by jet lag.

****

Hiram Fong retired from the United States Senate because the 9,116-mile airplane trip between his home in Hawaii and his office in Washington, D.C. was too debilitating. He traveled from Hawaii to work eighteen times a year and suffered from a chronic state of jet lag.

****

In *The Making of the Popes 1978*, author Andrew M. Greeley admitted that on his first day at his hotel in Rome, he felt he was "going to pieces." He had lost his glasses, walked out of the hotel without his wallet, forgotten phone numbers, and was in "mortal terror" of missing his appointments. Such was his state of jet lag.

****

In a death-bed interview, former Secretary of State John Foster Dulles admitted that he felt his decision on the controversial Aswan Dam in Egypt was one of the great mistakes of his life, and that he might have taken a more conciliatory stance with the Egyptians had he not been so weary from jet travel.

Jet lag has ruined more vacations, been the reason for more botched business meetings, and wreaked more general havoc on the air traveler than all the preflight or inflight irritations combined. Indeed, a term that four decades ago was an insider's expression used exclusively by an elite group of aviators, "jet lag" is now virtually a household word to 2.8 million passengers who have flown coast to coast in the United States, 2.1 million who have flown abroad from the United States, and more than 140 million people from around the globe who have flown through the world's international airports. Yet, despite the multitude of sufferers, only a handful of scientists specializing in chronobiology (the study of how time affects living organisms) and circadian regulatory biology (the study of how to control man's daily body rhythms) know its real cause, the true nature of its body-wide effect, and its simple cure.

The Phenomenon of East/West Flight

The biggest misconception that air travelers have is that jet lag is caused by being enclosed in a vehicle that is traveling at great speeds and at terrifically high altitudes. Somehow, air travelers correlate speed and altitude as key factors in jet lag. Yet the inflight velocity of the airplane and the distance traveled above the earth, *per se*, have absolutely nothing to do with jet lag. Nor do typical inflight symptoms of ear-popping, light headedness, dehydration, irritability, motion sickness, and any other ailment about which air travelers might complain while en route to their destination. All these problems can be attributed to poor cabin pressure, drinking alcoholic beverages while in flight, and nerve-wracking engine noises—not jet lag. Jet lag is strictly a phenomenon of long distance, east/west, too rapid travel to a new time frame.

The True Causes of Jet Lag: Disruption of Sense of Time, Sense of Place, and Sense of Well-Being

Every creature on earth is equipped with a wide variety of innate detection and measuring systems that are traditionally referred to as the five senses. These senses allow man to see, hear, feel, taste, and smell. Yet to scientists specializing in chronobiology and regulatory biology, three other more abstract, but equally important, "senses" exist: the sense of place, the sense of time, and, as a byproduct of both, the sense of well-being.

Sense of Place. All locations are physically, geographically, and even chemically different from one another either dramatically or subtly. Concomitantly, all living organisms have a keen sense of place and express it either consciously or unconsciously. In man, consciously it makes him homesick for familiar surroundings and wish for his own bed, and unconsciously he yearns for the accustomed hometown patterns of something as simple as the time frame of the sunrise and sunset. In other animals, like the salmon, it causes them to turn virtually mid-stream or mid-ocean to return to their place of origin.

Sense of Time. All people, animals, and plants have a natural ingrained sense of time and timing that is tied to sense of place. In man, every cell produces proteins and gene products on a preordained program that takes about a day to run, and senses the distinctive qualities of six in the morning, noon, and midnight. In other animals, as if a switch were thrown, it makes them change their course, migrate, store food, or hibernate. In plants, it causes the blossoms of the chrysanthemum to burst open one day and the flowers of the poinsettia yet another day.

Sense of Well-Being. Inextricably dependent on sense of time and sense of place is sense of well-being. An upheaval in the sense of time or sense of place, or both, precipitates a disruption in a person's sense of well-being.

For 250,000 years, man's sense of well-being, as related to sense of time and sense of place, was intact. Restrictions upon man's movements were imposed upon him by the pace he could set with his own feet, the speed and stamina of the animals that he domesticated and rode, the stroke of his canoe paddle, or his ability to build a sea-worthy vessel. He took weeks, months, years, or generations to travel great distances around the earth.

It was the advent of the propeller plane that ushered in a new era of increased mobility, and paved the way for a brand new phenomenon—jet lag. As the Wright brothers took to the air, geographic restrictions automatically placed on man as an earth-bound animal were lifted, and he attained the ability to "fly with the eagle," but not the corresponding travel instincts.

Those animals that developed the ability to fly or swim great distances have, during the course of evolution, become endowed with an ingrained set of instructions that prevent the animals from developing symptoms associated with rapid travel. The Canada goose, which flies literally thousands of miles each year during migration, listens to a kind of inner voice that limits the easterly or westerly range of flight. (Those few species of birds that do fly great distances in an easterly or westerly direction always rest for several days in one location before continuing their journey.) The gray whale swims the entire length of the West coast from Alaska to Mexico, yet if you chart his course, you will see that he, too, stays within a limited number of miles in an easterly or westerly direction, and swims, instead, much more north to south than east to west.

Not so nature's most highly evolved creature, man. He never developed the bird's inner voice or the whale's instinct to keep him traveling in the "proper" directions. Now, man soars encapsulated in a jet plane from east to west or west to east with an abandon beyond the wildest dreams of any winged or finned creature on earth. Yet, still possessed of essentially a Stone Age body that should be traveling great distances very, very slowly, if at all, he suffers the consequences in the form of jet lag.

The Chronobiological and Biochemical Basis of Jet Lag

The universe is filled with cycles within cycles within cycles. Each planet orbits the sun in an individual planetary year, 365 days for the planet earth. Within the earth's planetary year, there is a cycle of four seasons: spring, summer, fall, and winter. The moon, as it revolves around the earth, waxes and wanes in the light of the sun about every twenty-seven days.

As part of the cyclic universe, humans have their own cycles, many of which have been studied and charted by chronobiologists (scientists who specialize in cycles as they relate to living beings). These studies reveal that the human body is controlled by a master clock in the brain and inter-related satellite "time-keepers" throughout the body. Precision-timed and performing like clockwork, the satellites adjust and readjust, turn on and turn off, speed up and slow down all your biochemical processes throughout the day. In definite cyclical patterns, the time-keepers control your hormone levels, blood pressure, body temperature, digestive enzymes, kidneys, bladder, heart, brainwaves, etc., and see that all your internal systems are synchronized not only with one another, but with the cycles of your world as well.

The master clock and satellite time-keepers take their "cues" from several major sources in your immediate environment. The level of illumination, brightness of sunlight, and clock-time-of-day (external cues); food, drugs, and medication (internal cues); work, exercise, and periods of personal interaction (social cues) combine to lock in and reinforce your sense of time and sense of place, and they synchronize what is known to the scientific community as your circadian rhythms,* and to the lay reader as daily body rhythms.**

The synchronization of these rhythms is crucial and relies heavily on the presence of consistent daily patterns. Different time frames and unexpected cues are an anathema to body rhythms. When you virtually pitch yourself halfway around the globe, the unfamiliar timing requirements of the external, internal, and social cues around you at your flight destination set in motion a biochemical phase shift that marks the onslaught of jet lag. This shift triggers a major disruption in the synchronization of the time-keepers and body rhythms that keep your heart pumping to one beat while your lungs inhale and exhale to another, that put you to sleep at night and wake you in the morning, and that control the timing of every function of your body—right down to the level of a single cell.

When you board a jet plane and fly faster than the rotation of the earth or against the direction of its rotation, upon arrival you have to reset not only your wristwatch to reflect local time, but your entire twenty-four-hour biochemical schedule as well. It is this required shift that is at the root of jet lag.

After an easterly or westerly flight, the "hands" of the literally billions of body clocks that exist within the human body begin to, in a sense, spin as they search for a new schedule that will enable all your systems to function compatibly again. That interval of adjustment is described by scientists as a *transient state of dyschronism*. This is known commonly as jet lag and is that period of time during which the well-defined "old" body rhythms play tug-of-war with the still-to-be-defined "new" body rhythms that must develop as the body adapts to a different sense of time and place.

*As in *"circa* 1776, Paul Revere made silver," *circa* means "about"; *dian* comes from the Latin word *dies*, for "one day." *Circadian* therefore equals "about one day."

In the late 1940s, Franz Halberg, M.D., a professor at the University of Minnesota, coined the word "circadian" after he noticed rhythmic variations throughout the day in the count of white blood cells in laboratory animals.

**Not to be confused with "biorhythms," which have no scientific basis.

Of course, since jet lag occurs when you change time frames, it is strictly a phenomenon of time zones crossed during east/west flight. You can fly thousands of miles from Boston to Lima, Peru, and not experience jet lag; thousands of miles from Chicago to Mexico City and feel fine; and thousands of miles from Nome, Alaska, to Papeete, Tahiti—only an hour's difference—and adjust very quickly. When you travel in an essentially northerly or southerly direction, you do not change more than one or two time zones. When it is noon in Boston, it is also noon in Lima. Yes, you affect your "sense of place," but since your sense of time remains essentially undisturbed, your sense of well-being readjusts rapidly.

However, if you fly east/west from Bangor to Los Angeles and experience more than three hours time difference you can expect a bout of jet lag. Or, if you fly north/south from Chicago and combine it with an east/west angle that brings you to New Zealand—a six-hour difference—you can count on experiencing jet lag.

That is why jet lag commonly begins when you land and step out of the airplane, and not before. Jet lag starts when you have to adjust not only your wristwatch to reflect a different local time, but also your own daily internal biological rhythms of sleeping and waking, digestion and elimination, on the basis of a new time and new place.

Compounding the problem is that body rhythms exhibit a kind of lingering memory and resist change. In order to keep you running smoothly, they want to cling to the same old familiar schedule on the basis of the past time and place cues. The old rhythms corresponding to when the sun would have risen or set back home, when your alarm would have gone off, when you would have eaten, when you would have used the toilet and when you would have been working or socializing—each of these old rhythms persist tenaciously. Internal clocks still expect breakfast on the hometown schedule and prepare for it by releasing enzymes and stomach acids in anticipation of receiving food—yet no food may be eaten because although it is breakfast time back home, it is mid-afternoon in Paris when the airplane lands. Similarly, the internal clock is programmed to promote sleep on hometown time and consequently begins to "shut down"—even though the sun may just be rising in India when long-distance passengers disembark from the airplane; and the internal clock, programmed to keep the brain functioning optimally from early morning through the work day and into the evening in a hometown time frame, remains alert—even though jet travelers may just be emerging into total darkness at midnight in Japan.

To the air traveler, this transient state means only one thing: until your body can adapt to the new time frame, be it hours ahead or hours behind, jet lag will take its toll.

That's the bad news. The good news is that although body clocks are quite precise, like a spring-driven watch that can be reset, circadian dyschronism is a temporary state. Ultimately, the external, internal, and social cues at your flight destination will persuade the body clocks to reset themselves. The rise and set of the sun will exert an irresistible pressure on your body rhythms of sleep and wakefulness to "get in sync" with the new time frame, as it will when you eat your meals and when you socialize. In the interim you will experience a transient state of mental and physical "cellular" chaos—jet lag—as your body rhythms reluctantly begin to break their old daily patterns and shift to the new schedule in a new time frame.

The following is a list of human cycles—rapid, daily, weekly/monthly, yearly—that are disrupted by jet lag.

Cycles Disturbed by Jet Lag

Rapid ("Ultradian")	Daily ("Circadian")	Weekly/Monthly ("Infradian")	Yearly ("Circannual")

Heart
    heart beat
    pulse rate
	Heart
	    blood pressure
	    blood clotting
		Reproduction
		    ovulation
		    menstruation
		    hormone levels
			Life span
			    infancy
			    puberty
			    adulthood
			    old age

Lungs breathing	Eyesight		

Cell division	Mental ability
	    alertness
	    visual acuity
	    cognitive
	     function
			Reproduction
			    conception
			    birth
			    hormone levels

Eye blinking			
Swallowing			Cell replacement

Brain waves	Physical ability
	    physical prowess
	    energy levels
	    sense of pain		

	Sleep/wake		

	Digestion
	    bowel movements
	    urinary output
	    hunger pangs		

	Reproduction hormone levels		
	Temperature		
	Metabolism		
	Sense of time		
	Hair growth beard		

CHAPTER TWO

THE SYMPTOMS
OF JET LAG

If your trip has been in a north/south direction, and you feel tired when you leave the airplane, the problem is likely to be the garden variety of physical fatigue brought on by pressures associated with preparing for the trip—all the minutiae associated with finally being able to lock the front door and leave for the airport. In addition, having to lug suitcases, totebags, cameras, and briefcases to the car, bus, or train, as well as having to sit in a cramped position for however many hours you have been en route, will have taken a toll. All have conspired to leave you physically depleted when the airplane's wheels touch down. You will, however, recuperate as quickly as you can physically and mentally relax, because in north/south travel you do not change time zones, and therefore do not get jet lag.

The situation is not so easily remedied when you have undertaken an east/west flight. Although the same garden variety fatigue will be present for the exact same reasons after the flight, if you have not employed the Jet Lag Program, simple fatigue will soon be followed by a far more pervasive mental and physical debilitation.

Early Symptoms

Although it has been said that each traveler's physical and mental make-up is as individual as his fingerprints and therefore not everyone has every symptom that jet lag can produce, it is not unusual for people who have taken a long east/west flight to develop similar first-day symptoms of jet lag. These symptoms are far different from those that develop as a result of simply being tired, and without the Jet Lag Program they will not be remedied by a day of rest and recuperation.

Initially, on the first day at your destination, you begin to notice that you have an ever-growing sense of exhaustion that is far more pronounced than the general fatigue with which you left the airplane. It is an all-over, all-consuming weariness that affects your sense of time and place and well-being, as well as your concentration, memory, and performance.

What you are beginning to experience is very much like the situation you might have faced had you stayed home, but begun the "graveyard" shift at work for the first time in your life. Try as you might to shake off the fatigue, to concentrate, and to perform at your maximum capacity, you simply cannot.

Later Symptoms

Relentlessly, within hours of landing at your destination, the general fatigue and first-day early jet lag symptoms advance to an even more crushing level of enervation. Without the Jet Lag Program to reduce the severity of symptoms or eliminate them entirely, jet lag now produces significant gastrointestinal disorders of constipation or diarrhea, insomnia, loss of appetite, headache, impaired night vision, and limited peripheral vision. The symptoms become body-wide and often debilitating. To an athlete flying in from California a day or two before running in the New York City Marathon, jet lag means that he or she will be competing while, in a sense, physically and mentally handicapped in comparison to local athletes, whose body rhythms are running smoothly, or to those who have arrived early enough to have had time to adjust naturally and get over jet lag. Similarly, a couple just returning from a vacation in Amsterdam to Iowa will be putting themselves in a situation weighted toward trouble if quick reflexes and good vision are required during the drive from the airport to home; and a woman arriving in London from Bangor, Maine, who attempts to cross the street, may "forget" that traffic flows on the "wrong" side of the road in England and inadvertently step out into the street, having looked left when she should have looked right, and then not having had the rapid response time necessary to get out of the way of oncoming traffic.

Duration of Symptoms:
With and Without the Three-Step
Jet Lag Program

How long does it take for the body to readjust to a new time zone? In an effort to find out, international researchers have studied man and laboratory rats on both real and simulated jet flights around the world. By carefully monitoring body rhythms before departure, during flight, while at the destination, and after the return home, these researchers have been able to establish what normal body rhythms are, record how quickly and severely they are disrupted by a time change, and determine how long the symptoms of this disruption—or jet lag—lasts.

What scientists determined was that each person's body clock has its own adjustment rate. In other words, all body clocks do not shift simultaneously. Like a jewelry store display window that is filled with hundreds of functioning clocks, each of which is set to a different time, each individual cell in your body has its own clock, and each has its own alarm to signal daily functions—turning them down, up, or off—on different schedules throughout the day. When the shopkeeper steps into the window to turn all the clocks ahead or back, he can only get to so many so fast. Some alarms go off on the new schedule, while others continue on the old routine until the shopkeeper gets to them, too.

That is why on a trip that requires a five- to eight-hour time change (for example, a trip from the United States to Germany as illustrated in a comparison of fatigue symptoms **with** and **without** jet lag countermeasures), scientists have found it can take anywhere from two days to two weeks for sleep patterns to adjust thoroughly. Heart rate, which is normally faster in the day than at night, can take from five to six days to synchronize. Urinary output, which generally decreases during the night, can take up to ten days to normalize. The gastrointestinal system, which controls the bowels, can take twenty-four hours per time zone crossed before elimination routines readjust. Reactions to light signals, grip strength, and ability to calculate mathematical problems can take from two days to nearly two weeks to straighten out. Elementary psychomotor performance (coordination and reflexes) can take from five to ten days to recover.

The following is a list of jet lag symptoms that begin immediately upon deplaning.

Early and Late Jet Lag Symptoms

Early Symptoms	Late Symptoms
fatigue	constipation or diarrhea
disorientation	lack of sexual interest
reduced physical ability	limited peripheral vision
reduced mental acuity	decreased muscle tone
confusion	impaired night vision
upset appetite	reduced physical work capacity
off-schedule bowel and urinary movements	disrupted phases of body rhythms and functions
onset of memory loss	slowed response time to visual stimulation
	reduced motor coordination and reflex time
	interference with prescription drugs
	insomnia
	acute fatigue
	loss of appetite
	headache

DEGREE OF FATIGUE EXPERIENCED AFTER FLIGHT FROM KANSAS TO GERMANY, WITH AND WITHOUT THE JET LAG PROGRAM.

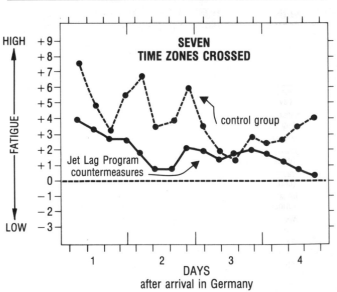

The following two figures indicate the degree of time required to resynchronize specific body functions **without** the Jet Lag Program to eliminate symptoms (short trips) or greatly reduce them (long trips).

Typical resynchronization periods (in days) after time zone changes (<u>without</u> the use of the Three-Step Jet Lag Program)
EASTBOUND FLIGHTS

	Time Zone Change (in hours)					
	2 hours	4 hours	6 hours	8 hours	10 hours	12 hours
Performance (psychomotor)	3	6–7	9–10	12	12	12 +
Reaction time (vigilance)	1–2	3–4	5	6–7	8	8
Heart rate	2	4	6	8	8–10	8–10
Corticosteroids (urinary)	4	7–8	11–12	12	12	12 +
Noradrenaline (urinary)	1	2	3	4	4–5	4–5
Adrenaline (urinary)	2	4	6	8	8–10	8–10
Bowel movements	3	6–7	9–10	12	12	12 +
Body temperature	3	6	9	12	12	12 +
Sleep pattern	1	3–4	4–5	6–7	8–9	8–9

Typical resynchronization periods (in days) after time zone changes (<u>without</u> the use of the Three-Step Jet Lag Program)
WESTBOUND FLIGHTS

	Time Zone Change (in hours)					
	2 hours	4 hours	6 hours	8 hours	10 hours	12 hours
Performance (psychomotor)	2	4	6	8	10	12 +
Reaction time (vigilance)	1	1–2	2–3	3	4	5–8
Heart rate	1–2	2–3	4	5–6	6–7	8–10
Corticosteroids (urinary)	2–3	5	7–8	10–11	12	12 +
Noradrenaline (urinary)	1	1–2	2	2–3	3–4	4–5
Adrenaline (urinary)	1–2	2–3	4	5–6	6–7	8–10
Bowel movements	2–3	4–5	7	9	11	12 +
Body temperature	2	4	6	8	10	12 +
Sleep pattern	1	2	3–4	4–5	6–7	8–9

How effective is the Three-Step Jet Lag Program? Take a look at the two figures below. As you can see, the Jet Lag Program can have a profound effect on the severity and duration of jet lag symptoms, and can, in fact, eliminate them altogether on the less extreme time zone changes.

General comparison (in days) of duration of symptoms with and without the Three-Step Jet Lag Program
EASTBOUND FLIGHTS

Time Zone Changes	With Jet Lag Program*	Without Jet Lag Program
+2	0	3
+4	0	6
+6	1	9
+8	2	12
+10	3	12
+12	3	12+

*Jet lag symptoms experienced while on the Jet Lag Program will be greatly reduced in potential severity.

General comparison (in days) of duration of symptoms with and without the Three-Step Jet Lag Program
WESTBOUND FLIGHTS

Time Zone Changes	With Jet Lag Program*	Without Jet Lag Program
−2	0	2
−4	0	4
−6	1	6
−8	1	8
−10	2	10
−12	3	12+

*Jet lag symptoms experienced while on the Jet Lag Program will be greatly reduced in potential severity.

During the course of their investigation, scientists also discovered that, although the Three-Step Jet Lag Program can dramatically decrease the overall period of adjustment on long trips and even eliminate it on very short trips, jet lag symptoms can also be affected by a myriad of seemingly disparate factors, including number of time zones through which you pass, personality, eating habits, and, surprisingly, the nature of social or business pressures that force you to get up and get going.

What follows is a breakdown of factors beyond the reach of the Jet Lag Program that can affect the duration of symptoms experienced by air travelers.

Time Zone Factors

Long Haul versus Short Haul. Obviously, the more time zones through which you pass, the more severe the body clock upheaval and jet lag symptoms. If you fly halfway around the world, your jet lag symptoms will be much more severe and last much longer than if you opt for a trip that is a quarter as long.

Also, recovery from a westbound trip is in fact from 30% to 50% swifter than from an eastbound one. Although no one is quite certain why east to west flights cause less circadian rhythm disruption than west to east flights, it is *surmised* that "gaining" time, rather than "losing" time, is easier for the human body to handle. A handy way to re-member this east to west phenomenon is contained in the words of the American writer Horace Greeley, who is re-nowned for his advice to the youth of his day to "go west young man, go west."

Personality Factors

Evening versus Daytime. Many people describe them-selves as "morning" types. They are able to leap out of bed, get dressed, and get going even while "night" types are rising and falling back into bed three times prior to actually getting up. When it comes to jet lag, it is the night owl who seems to fare better when traveling in a westerly direction, rather than the morning lark, and vice versa in an east-erly direction. According to Drs. K. E. Klein and H. M. Wegmann of the West German Institute for Aviation Med-icine, this is because "evening types seem not to experience sleep deficiency, and more easily extend the sleep period when sleep onset is shifted to late hours."

Extrovert versus Introvert. If you are gregarious and enjoy talking, mixing with people, and doing things in a group, you are less likely to experience severe jet lag than a fellow traveler who retreats to his room upon arrival, prefers to see the sights alone, eats supper by himself, and generally leads a more reclusive existence. Exposing your-self to outside visual and mental stimuli causes chemical changes to take place in your brain to help keep you more alert.

Regimented versus Flexible. Some people live by the clock. They get up when the alarm goes off, eat a snack at precisely the same time every morning, head out for lunch at exactly lunchtime, have supper on the table at the same time every night, and retire without fail right after the late night news. Other people prefer to rise at varying times, depending on the requirements of the daily schedule, eat snacks and main meals only when hunger pangs arise, and call it a day only when they actually feel like going to sleep. Of these two types, the more regimented personality will experience less jet lag. Accustomed to doing things "by the clock," this type marches more readily to a new circadian beat.

Stable versus Neurotic. Anxious people secrete hormones and neurotransmitters that unsettle body rhythms. Therefore, the less easily frazzled you are by circumstance, the more easily you will adapt to a new time zone. If you are keyed up all the time, your body rhythms will have a more difficult time adjusting to an entirely new schedule.

Social Factors
Pressured versus Relaxed. If you simply cannot give in to jet lag symptoms because you need to attend an important meeting, give a concert performance, compete in a contest or make it to another airplane, bus, or train on time, the demands of the situation may enable you to rise above jet lag, perhaps not totally, but at least temporarily. Despite the presence of jet lag, by dint of will you can force yourself to function to the best of your ability and thereby accomplish much more than if you surrendered to jet lag without a fight. Once you begin to function, other factors, such as environmental and social cues, combine to help you maintain your level of activity.

Age Factors
Youth versus Middle Age versus Old Age. Although the very young may not appear to their parents to experience jet lag, they do. Infants' body rhythms are actually heavily involved in waking/sleeping cycles; for example, their pattern just happens to be not that of adults. However, infants adjust more rapidly than older people.

Body rhythm patterns are based loosely on the twelve daylight hours and twelve nighttime hours. When people of middle age—neither young nor old—experience a time zone change, jet lag sets in, but it is overcome as the old light/dark pattern eventually gives way to a shifted pattern.

Possibly because of weakened or exhausted internal timesetters produced by the aging process, the elderly suffer the most severe form of jet lag. Body rhythms of the aged tend to be already in a process of slipping out of synchronization with the twelve/twelve pattern and into "circadian desynchronization."

If you are elderly and leading an increasingly more sedentary life, you may have noticed that your sleep patterns have altered significantly since middle age. Part of this is compensation for a less demanding schedule. You no longer require as much sleep, and often, when it comes, it is fragmented. (In fact, by age sixty-five, 40% of men and women have difficulty sleeping.) When the elderly change time zones, they are asking an already disrupted system to experience greater upheaval, and then to adjust and stabilize. Eventually, jet lag will subside, but it will have taken an unusually severe toll. However, a hidden benefit of severe jet lag and the resultant reestablishment of a new body rhythm in a new time zone is often a sense of renewed vigor and a sudden ability to sleep through the night. For this reason, the Three-Step Jet Lag Program can be particularly advantageous to the elderly. Through the Three-Step Program, not only are jet lag symptoms reduced, but the program literally forces a resynchronization that might otherwise have eluded the elderly person for years, if not for the rest of his/her life.

Health Factors

Good Health versus Illness. If you are in ill-health, jet lag may make you feel even worse. Sickness and disease cause their own disruption of body rhythms, and jet lag compounds the feeling of malaise. There is good evidence that disrupted body rhythms permit or encourage or even cause illness, particularly mental illness in the category of "affective disorders" and depression.

Drugs versus No Drugs. If you are taking prescription or nonprescription drugs, often the timing of these drugs is crucial to their working properly. When you change time zones, your body clock begins to adjust accordingly. As a result, drugs can temporarily lose their effectiveness or even have a detrimental effect, depending upon at what point they are taken during the twenty-four-hour day. At the University of Minnesota, the effectiveness of chemotherapy has been proved to depend significantly upon what time of day the drugs are administered.

Even such ubiquitous drugs as alcohol, nicotine, marijuana, and coffee cause changes in your biochemistry that disrupt your body rhythms throughout the day and night. Taken alone or in combination, they can worsen the problem of jet lag and jet lag recuperation.

All this means that it is very difficult to be specific about the length of time required to adapt to a new time zone. It depends upon: (1) how many time zones you have crossed, (2) whether you have flown from west to east or from east to west, (3) what personality, social, age, and health factors are involved, and (4) whether you have employed any counter-measures, such as described in the Three-Step Jet Lag Program, before, during, and after the trip.

Also, some people are better endowed genetically than others with flexible body clocks that can be readily reset, either forward or backward. Furthermore, in the course of a trip, some people inadvertently do all of the "wrong" things to counteract jet lag, while others, the lucky ones, accidentally hit upon the "right" things to do to respond to the challenge.

CHAPTER THREE

A LESSON IN TIME

The Time Structure of the Environment

Briefly stated, the present system uses twenty-four standard meridians of longitude (imaginary lines on the earth's surface that run from the North Pole to the South Pole), each fifteen degrees apart, starting with the "prime" meridian at Greenwich, England, which accounts for what is called Greenwich Mean Time.

Meridians are superimposed lines that divide the earth into twenty-four standard time zones. In practice, the boundaries of some time zones zig-zag for the convenience of local residents, and at the discretion of some city planners. For the most part, however, time is uniform throughout an individual time zone, and with just a few exceptions, each time zone differs from the ones it borders by exactly an hour.

Due to the earth's rotation, daylight travels from one meridian to the next in a westerly direction for a total of twenty-four meridians during the course of a twenty-four-hour day. During eastbound travel, the day shortens; that is, the clock must be set ahead for as many hours as the number of time zones that have been crossed. Similarly, during westbound travel, the clock has to be set back.

The Ribbons of Cities table provides an extremely accurate reference to determine the north/south or east/west direction of flights. It is based strictly on longitude. If you want to travel in a direction that makes the Three-Step Jet Lag Program virtually unnecessary, fly more north/south than east/west. Should your trip involve a significant east/west route, however, you must implement the Three-Step Jet Lag Program in order to dramatically reduce or even eliminate jet lag symptoms.

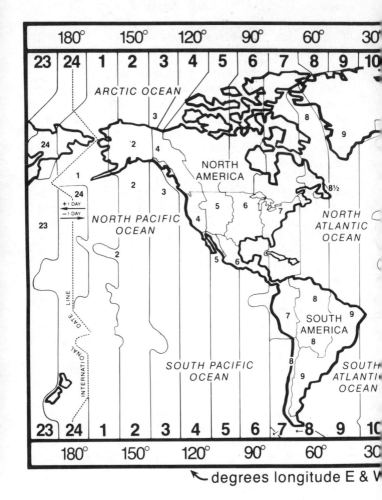

MERCATOR MAP. TIME ZONES OF THE WORLD

The Mercator Map has been the standard navigation map for centuries. Because of its distinctive design, with polar regions exaggerated, it is an indispensible aid for jet travelers counting the number of time zone changes involved in flight.

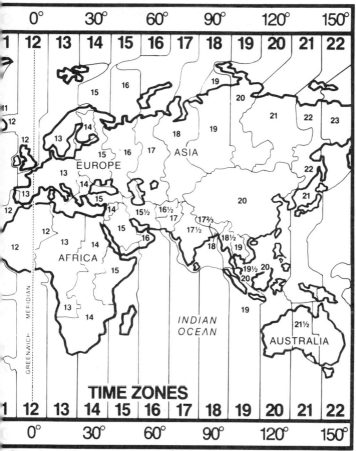

TIME ZONES

Greenwich Meridian ↗

RIBBONS OF CITIES—
LOCATION OF LANDMARK CITIES
ACCORDING TO WORLD TIME ZONES

STD TIME ZONES IDL*	1h
STD TIME ZONES GMT**	−11h
	WESTERN ALASKA

NAME OF TIME ZONE	WAST
APPROXIMATE*** BASIC	
LONGITUDE (W-E)	165°W

ARCTIC CIRCLE

| 66.5°N LAT | NOME |
| | DUTCH HARBOR |

TROPIC OF CANCER

23.5°N LAT

— EQUATOR 0°N LAT —————————————

| | PAGO PAGO |
| | (Samoa) |

23.5°S LAT

TROPIC OF CAPRICORN

66.5°S LAT

ANTARCTIC CIRCLE

* Standard time zones 1–24, with reference to the International Date Line.
** Standard time zones 1–24, with reference to Greenwich Mean Time.
*** As discussed earlier, in some cases cities are in a time zone removed
from the expected longitude, due to local preference; these are
shown by L− or −L, symbolizing direction of the true longitude.

2h −10h ALASKA–HAWAII	3h −9h WEST YUKON	4h −8h PACIFIC
AHST	WYST	PST
150°W	135°W	120°W
BARROW		
FAIRBANKS ANCHORAGE		JUNEAU VANCOUVER SEATTLE PORTLAND SAN FRANCISCO LOS ANGELES SAN DIEGO
HONOLULU		
PAPEETE L − (Tahiti)		

RIBBONS OF CITIES—
LOCATION OF LANDMARK CITIES
ACCORDING TO WORLD TIME ZONES

STD TIME ZONES IDL*	5h	6h
STD TIME ZONES GMT**	−7h	−6h
	MOUNTAIN	CENTRAL
NAME OF TIME ZONE	MST	CST
APPROXIMATE*** BASIC		
LONGITUDE (W-E)	105°W	90°W

ARCTIC CIRCLE

66.5°N LAT	EDMONTON	WINNIPEG
	CALGARY	MINNEAPOLIS
		OMAHA
	SALT LAKE CITY	CHICAGO
	DENVER	KANSAS CITY
	PHOENIX	DALLAS-FT. WORTH
		HOUSTON
		NEW ORLEANS

TROPIC OF CANCER

23.5°N LAT		MEXICO CITY
		GUATEMALA

— EQUATOR 0°N LAT —

23.5°S LAT

TROPIC OF CAPRICORN

66.5°S LAT

ANTARCTIC CIRCLE

*Standard time zones 1–24, with reference to the International Date Line.
**Standard time zones 1–24, with reference to the Greenwich Mean Time.
***As discussed earlier, in some cases cities are in a time zone removed
from the expected longitude, due to local preference; these are
shown by L− or −L, symbolizing direction of the true longitude.

7h −5h EASTERN	8h −4h ATLANTIC	9h −3h ARGENTINE and E. BRAZILIAN
EST	AST	ABST
75°W	60°W	45°W
	SONDRE STROMFJORD	
MONTREAL TORONTO BOSTON DETROIT CLEVELAND NEW YORK PHILADELPHIA WASHINGTON-BALTIMORE ATLANTA TAMPA MIAMI NASSAU	HALIFAX HAMILTON (Bermuda)	
KINGSTON (Jamaica) HAVANA PANAMA CITY BOGOTA	SAN JUAN, P.R. CARACAS FORT-DE-FRANCE (Martinique)	
QUITO LIMA	LA PAZ	BRASILIA RIO DE JANEIRO
	SANTIAGO DE CHILE	SAO PAOLO MONTEVIDEO BUENOS AIRES

RIBBONS OF CITIES—
LOCATION OF LANDMARK CITIES
ACCORDING TO WORLD TIME ZONES

	10h	11h
STD TIME ZONES IDL*		
STD TIME ZONES GMT**	−2h	−1
	MIDATLANTIC	AZORES
NAME OF TIME ZONE	MAST	AST
APPROXIMATE*** BASIC		
LONGITUDE (W-E)	30°W	15°W
		SCORESBYSUND
ARCTIC CIRCLE		(Greenland)

66.5°N LAT

SANTA MARIA.
(Azores)

TROPIC OF CANCER

23°N LAT

— EQUATOR 0°N LAT —

FERNANDO
DE NORONHA
(Brazil)

23.5°S LAT

TROPIC OF CAPRICORN

66.5°S LAT

ANTARCTIC CIRCLE

*Standard time zones 1–24, with reference to the International Date Line.
**Standard time zones 1–24, with reference to Greenwich Mean Time.
***As discussed earlier, in some cases cities are in a time zone removed
from the expected longitude, due to local preference; these are
shown by L− or −L, symbolizing direction of the true longitude.

12h	13h	14h
0h	+ 1h	+ 2h
GREENWICH	CENTRAL	BALKAN EGYPT
GMT	CET	BEST
0	15°E	30°E

REYKJAVIK	OSLO	HELSINKI
LONDON	STOCKHOLM	BUCHAREST
DUBLIN	COPENHAGEN	SOFIA
LISBON	BERLIN	ATHENS
CASABLANCA	WARSAW	BEIRUT
ALGIERS	AMSTERDAM	TEL AVIV
LOS PALMAS	BRUSSELS	CAIRO
(Canary Islands)	LUXEMBOURG	
	FRANKFURT, PRAGUE	
	PARIS, MUNICH	
	VIENNA, GENEVA	
	ZURICH	
	MILAN	
	ROME, BELGRADE	
	MADRID	
	TUNIS	

DAKAR	LAGOS	KHARTOUM
ACCRA		

	BRAZZAVILLE	

		JOHANNESBURG
		CAPE TOWN

RIBBONS OF CITIES—
LOCATION OF LANDMARK CITIES
ACCORDING TO WORLD TIME ZONES

STD TIME ZONES IDL*	15h	16h
STD TIME ZONES GMT**	+3h	+4h
	MOSCOW-ARABIA- E. AFRICA TIME	BAKU-ABU DHABI TIME
NAME OF TIME ZONE	MEAT	BAT
APPROXIMATE*** BASIC		
LONGITUDE (W-E)	45°E	60°E
ARCTIC CIRCLE	MURMANSK	
66.5°N LAT	LENINGRAD	KAZAN
	MOSCOW	VOLGOGRAD
	KIEV	BAKU
	ANKARA	ABU DHABI
	ISTANBUL TEHERAN 3½	
	BAGHDAD	
	KUWAIT	
	DHARAN	

TROPIC OF CANCER

23.5°N LAT	JIDDAH ADDIS ABABA	

EQUATOR 0°N LAT	NAIROBI DAR ES SALAAM	

23.5°S LAT

TROPIC OF CAPRICORN

66.5°S LAT

ANTARCTIC CIRLE

*Standard time zones 1–24, with reference to the International Date Line.
**Standard time zones 1–24, with reference to Greenwich Mean Time.
***As discussed earlier, in some cases cities are in a time zone removed
from the expected longitude, due to local preference; these are
shown by L− or −L, symbolizing direction of the true longitude.

17h +5h KARACHI TIME	18h +6h OMSK TIME	19h +7h BANGKOK TIME
KT	OT	BT
75°E	90°E	105°E

SVERDLOVSK KARACHI	DELHI 5½ OMSK TASHKENT	NOVOSIBIRSK

KABUL 4½

CALCUTTA 5½ BOMBAY 5½ COLOMBO 5½	RANGOON 6½	BANGKOK

		JAKARTA

RIBBONS OF CITIES—
LOCATION OF LANDMARK CITIES
ACCORDING TO WORLD TIME ZONES

STD TIME ZONES IDL*	20h	21h
STD TIME ZONES GMT**	+8h	+9h
	PEKING	JAPAN
	SHANGHAI	STANDARD
	TIME	TIME
NAME OF TIME ZONE	PST	JST
APPROXIMATE*** BASIC		
LONGITUDE (W-E)	120°E	135°E

ARCTIC CIRCLE

66.5°N LAT	IRKUTSK	
	PEKING	
	LHASA	TOKYO
	SHANGHAI	SEOUL

TROPIC OF CANCER

23.5°N LAT	HONG KONG
	MANILA
	SINGAPORE

— EQUATOR 0°N LAT —————————————————

23.5°S LAT

TROPIC OF CAPRICORN   PERTH

66.5°S LAT

ANTARCTIC CIRCLE

*Standard time zones 1–24, with reference to the International Date Line.
**Standard time zones 1–24, with reference to Greenwich Mean Time.
***As discussed earlier, in some cases cities are in a time zone removed
from the expected longitude, due to local preference; these are
shown by L– or –L, symbolizing direction of the true longitude.

22h	23h	24h
+10h	+11h	+12h
SYDNEY	TRUK	NEW
MELBOURNE	TIME	ZEALAND
TIME		TIME
SMT	TT	NZT
150°E	165°E	180°E

		KAMCHATSKIY
VLADIVOSTOK		

GUAM	TRUK	WAKE

DARWIN 9½	PORT MORESBY	NOUMÉA (New Caledonia)	FIJI

ADELAIDE 9½	SYDNEY MELBOURNE		AUCKLAND WELLINGTON

The following figure displays time zone changes from the United States ONLY to eighty different countries around the world. Determine whether the city from which you are departing the United States is on eastern, central, mountain or pacific standard time; then find your destination city along the left hand column.

TIME DIFFERENCES BETWEEN STANDARD U.S. TIME ZONES (EASTERN, CENTRAL, MOUNTAIN AND PACIFIC STANDARD TIMES) AND FOREIGN COUNTRIES.

| | TIME DIFFERENCE U.S. TIME ZONE | | |
	EST	CST	MST	PST
American Samoa	−6	−5	−4	−3
Andorra	6	7	8	9
Argentina	2	3	4	5
Australia	16	17	18	19
Austria	6	7	8	9
Bahrain	8	9	10	11
Belgium	6	7	8	9
Belize	−1	0	1	2
Bolivia	1	2	3	4
Brazil	2	3	4	5
Chile	2	3	4	5
Colombia	0	1	2	3
Costa Rica	−1	0	1	2
Cyprus	7	8	9	10
Denmark	6	7	8	9
Ecuador	0	1	2	3
El Salvador	−1	0	1	2
Fiji	17	18	19	20
Finland	7	8	9	10
France	6	7	8	9
French Antilles	1	2	3	4
Germany	6	7	8	9

	TIME DIFFERENCE U.S. TIME ZONE			
	EST	CST	MST	PST
Greece	7	8	9	10
Guam	15	16	17	18
Guatemala	−1	0	1	2
Guyana	2	3	4	5
Haiti	0	1	2	3
Honduras	−1	0	1	2
Hong Kong	13	14	15	16
Indonesia (Western)	12	13	14	15
Iran	8½	9½	10½	11½
Iraq	8	9	10	11
Ireland	5	6	7	8
Israel	7	8	9	10
Italy	6	7	8	9
Ivory Coast	5	6	7	8
Japan	14	15	16	17
Kenya	8	9	10	11
Korea	14	15	16	17
Kuwait	8	9	10	11
Liberia	5	6	7	8
Libya	6	7	8	9
Liechtenstein	6	7	8	9
Luxembourg	6	7	8	9
Malaysia	13	14	15	16
Monaco	6	7	8	9
Netherlands	6	7	8	9
Netherlands Antilles	1	2	3	4
New Caledonia	16	17	18	19
New Zealand	17	18	19	20
Nicaragua	−1	0	1	2

	TIME DIFFERENCE U.S. TIME ZONE			
	EST	CST	MST	PST
Nigeria	6	7	8	9
Norway	6	7	8	9
Panama	0	1	2	3
Papua New Guinea	15	16	17	18
Paraguay	1	2	3	4
Peru	0	1	2	3
Philippines	13	14	15	16
Portugal	5	6	7	8
Romania	7	8	9	10
San Marino	6	7	8	9
Saudi Arabia	8	9	10	11
Senegal	5	6	7	8
Singapore	13	14	15	16
South Africa	7	8	9	10
Spain	6	7	8	9
Sri Lanka	10½	11½	12½	13½
Suriname	1½	2½	3½	4½
Sweden	6	7	8	9
Switzerland	6	7	8	9
Tahiti	−5	−4	−3	−2
Taiwan	13	14	15	16
Thailand	12	13	14	15
Tunisia	6	7	8	9
Turkey	8	9	10	11
U.S.S.R. (Eastern)	8	9	10	11
United Arab Emirates	9	10	11	12
United Kingdom	5	6	7	8
Venezuela	1	2	3	4
Yugoslavia	6	7	8	9

## CHAPTER FOUR

TRICKING BODY CLOCKS

Old Remedies versus the Three-Step Jet Lag Program

Many people simply do not have the luxury of allowing jet lag to diminish gradually over a period of days or weeks. Sometimes the duration of a trip is only a day or two, or a week, and jet lag symptoms can take so long to subside naturally that you may well be on your way home or about to take off for yet another destination before you have even adjusted to the new time zone in which you have landed.

In particular, the problem of jet lag concerns men and women who, for a variety of reasons, must be mentally sharp and/or physically fit almost, if not immediately, upon arrival. Often these people are diplomats who must negotiate sensitive issues with far-reaching implications; or athletes whose competitors include not only others suffering from jet lag, but local athletes at their peak of physical prowess; or business people for whom a convention or a specific meeting may be absolutely crucial to success or failure. For these people, uncontrolled jet lag presents a very serious situation.

Over the course of the years, however, a few "home" remedies have evolved, some no more than nonsensical or counterproductive, others more successful and useful because they accidentally incorporate helpful techniques. None, however, are as effective as the Three-Step Jet Lag Program.

The first remedy involves a preflight adjustment over a period of days before departure:

1. The Henry Kissinger Approach. When former Secretary of State Henry Kissinger knew he had to attend an important meeting in a foreign country, in the hope that he could systematically shift his body clocks to foreign time before he actually boarded the airplane, he would try to retire one hour earlier each night and rise one hour later.

Did it work? The problem with the Kissinger approach to "shuttle diplomacy" is that the demands of public and private life at home and before departure seldom permit the kind of rigid commitment and self-discipline this technique entails. Not only is it extremely difficult, as well as impractical, to withdraw so totally from daily events, it is actually impossible to remain unaffected physiologically by environmental influences such as the light/dark patterns and the social cues around you. If the technique worked at all, it did not work well. From the studies performed on phase shifts associated with body clock changes, in all likelihood Kissinger would experience nearly as much jet lag on the first day at his destination as the person who had sat next to him in the airplane.

The second approach involves arriving several days ahead of time when an important appointment, meeting, or event is scheduled:

2. The Dwight D. Eisenhower Approach. Former President Eisenhower, in 1955, flew into Geneva on a Friday for a summit meeting with Nikita Khrushchev the following Monday. Eisenhower had arrived early in order to try to reduce his jet lag symptoms in time for the meeting.

Was Eisenhower successful in reducing his jet lag symptoms? Partially, but not totally. Studies on jet lag symptoms indicate that recuperation actually does take about a day (more or less) per time zone through which the traveler has flown. Had Eisenhower arrived in Geneva an entire week prior to the summit meeting, he would have been well on his way to recovery, but in the absence of the other jet lag countermeasures discussed later, just two or three days are ordinarily not enough time for full adjustment to the new time zone. In fact, Eisenhower was still very much in a state of cellular upheaval, although his sleeping/waking patterns may have begun to synchronize with local time.

As an interesting note, companies such as Continental Oil and Phillips Petroleum have actually insisted that their executives use a modified Eisenhower approach and take one full day to adjust from easterly trips before resuming business-oriented activities. However, as in-depth studies have indicated, jet lag begins from the moment the plane lands and continues for days thereafter whenever a time zone change has occurred.

The third approach to jet lag is to adhere rigorously to your own hometown schedule, no matter where you are in the world:

3. The Lyndon Johnson Approach. Former President Johnson rarely, if ever, reset his wristwatch when Air Force One landed in a foreign country. When he flew to Guam to confer with President Nguyen Van Thieu of South Vietnam, Johnson remained on his usual time schedule, eating when he would have at the White House, sleeping when it was dark in Washington, D.C., and arranging meetings at his convenience during what were reasonable hours in the United States.

Was Johnson's technique effective? To a degree, yes, but his approach required an iron will and total denial of events transpiring around him. If you are interested in experiencing the country you are visiting by dining out, by touring its museums, etc., forcing yourself to remain on hometown time will put you totally out of sync with everyone else and everyone else's schedule.

If you schedule meetings at what might be the middle of the night at your destination, but only afternoon by your hometown schedule, will you be more alert? Yes, and perhaps you can get away with it if you are the President of the United States—but chances are other members of the meeting may not be willing to adjust their entire schedule to accommodate you.

The fourth way to control jet lag involves the systematic and orderly introduction of environmental cues and other agents that predictably influence body clocks; these include illumination, exercise, social cues, foods that encourage sleep, and common beverages that contain chemicals that trigger an amazing biochemical adjustment to a new time zone:

4. The Three-Step Jet Lag Approach. Beginning from one to three days prior to flight (depending on the number of time zones to be crossed) the Jet Lag Program continues for the day of the flight, and is ended after the first full day at your destination.

Will it be more effective than the other three approaches? Absolutely! And:

- You do not have to readjust your waking and sleeping patterns while at home by using the "Kissinger" technique for days prior to flight;
- You do not have to waste valuable vacation or business time recuperating for days from jet lag in a foreign hotel;

- You are better able to function from the moment you land because the program encourages you to step right into the mainstream of activity;
- You initiate the resetting and resynchronization of those body clocks that may have been disturbed prior to your actual trip;
- You feel fine before, during, and after your trip.

Finally, being informed about the basic causes and symptoms of jet lag, you are better equipped to deal with and to prevent the onset of similar problems and disorders in your daily living even when you are not engaged in global travel.

The Origins of the Jet Lag Program

For hundreds of years, researchers have studied a variety of the rhythms present in the universe and on earth, but only in the past few decades have scientists become concerned with how to force the rhythms of human body clocks ahead or back.

Years ago, with few exceptions, the need to alter body clocks simply did not exist. You lived life mostly in synchronization with the rhythms of nature. With the advent of candles, kerosene lamps, and, eventually, electric lights, these rhythms could be ignored to some extent but generally speaking, as members of a rural society, people stuck to the daytime (or diurnal) patterns and left the nights to the owls, bats, and other nocturnal creatures of the earth.

World War, twenty-four-hour security watches, around-the-clock assembly line work, and varying twenty-four-hour shifts for doctors, nurses, firemen, policemen, etc. (groups which now comprise easily 20% of the industrial world's work force) began to "turn night into day," and workers started to try to buck the daytime genetic programming of hundreds of millions of years of evolution. The result was greatly diminished mental acuity, enormous reduction in physical prowess that changed "sure win" to "sure lose," significant increases in errors and inefficiency, and the production of such overwhelming fatigue that workers often fell asleep on the job (all symptoms common among jet travelers who, by changing time zones, experience large body clock shifts as well).

The challenge fell to the scientists and researchers who, often with laboratory animals, but sometimes with humans as well, began not only to establish what normal daytime rhythms were, but also to try to determine ways to help turn a daytime creature into a nighttime animal, so that work could be performed more efficiently, and the number of problems associated with "shift work" would be eliminated or reduced.

The simpler studies performed were with animals under controlled conditions in laboratories. Some important preliminary research suggested that, since the daily rhythms of all body functions fluctuate in patterns throughout a twenty-four- or twenty-five-hour day, body temperature (which is higher in the day and lower at night) could provide one of the easiest and clearest indications of when body rhythms were in a state of transition and when they had finally assumed a daytime pattern during nighttime hours. Because temperature was known to be one of the last functions to complete a shift, it was safe to assume that when that shift had been made, all other body rhythms had shifted as well.

Once it was determined how many hours, days, and weeks were involved in the natural smoothing of disrupted body rhythms after a time shift, scientists were able to move on to an even more challenging aspect of body clocks—how to accelerate the shift artificially.

Light/Dark Phases, Food, Social Cues. Working with laboratory animals and humans, scientists first considered external factors that appeared to influence the body's clocks to become active or inactive. Although now there is a whole laundry list of known influences on body clocks, at the time there were only two. Designated as *zeitgebers* (pronounced *tsight-gaybers*, from the German for "time-givers"), they were the sunlight cue in cycles of light and darkness that "told" the man or animal when it was time to wake or when it was time to sleep, and the food cue that relieved hunger and supplied reserves of energy. However, a third cue, heretofore unsuspected, which influenced alertness and wakefulness, also existed.

This "social" cue involved the schedule of when the man or animal was used to getting up (whether by an alarm clock going off or having a laboratory technician turn the light switch on), when it would normally be performing its daytime tasks (working a job or running a maze), and when it would typically be interacting with others (conversing with the family in the evening or keeping contact until the technician turned out the lights). Social cues include interpersonal interaction, eating together rather than alone, and by extention, intense intellectual activity, homework and reading or writing—anything that involves **mental** stimulation.

Timing. Knowing that a phase shift is essentially a body-wide *biochemical event*, chronobiologists took the investigation yet another step. They discovered two facts: one, that your entire body chemistry changes over the course of a day, and that you are quite literally a different person biochemically at six in the morning than you are at midnight, so much so that it is the equivalent of being a redhead at dawn and a blond at midnight; and, two, because of this constant inconstancy within you, your body chemistry reacts quite differently at different times of the day to the same stimulus, ranging from not reacting at all, to reacting as expected, to reacting as if under acute stress.

Consider, for example, daylight as a cue to help set the body's timers and keep them in synchronization. How pleasant it is, how reinforcing to a sense of personal well-being, to soak up the sun's rays on a sunny beach. Mankind accepts light and takes pleasure in its presence during the *active phase* of his daily cycle, and rejects it and finds it abhorrent if it suddenly flashes on at three o'clock in the morning during his *inactive phase*. In humans, daytime exercise in the form of jogging, tennis, handball, swimming, and aerobic dancing are invigorating and positive reinforcers of body clocks during daytime activity, but an activity 180 degrees out of phase with "daytime" would be genuinely stressful.

Natural Chemicals. The search continued into man-made, as well as natural, drugs and chemicals that might also be combined with light and dark, food, and social "cues" to affect body rhythms. At this point another important discovery was made. It was found that a variety of chemicals, including those found quite naturally in beverages people were drinking every day, could act "chronobiotically," and dramatically speed up or slow down body clocks, depending upon at what time of day they were consumed and upon the speed with which they were consumed.

As explained in detail in the next chapter, the following is a "laundry list" of major influences on body clocks. With the exception of the drugs (the Jet Lag Program is drug-free) a combination of light and dark, food, physical and mental activities, methylated xanthines, and social interaction will play a major role in combating jet lag symptoms.

MAJOR INFLUENCES ON BODY CLOCKS

Light and dark
   sunlight
   electric lights
   window blinds

Food
   proteins
   carbohydrates
   fats

Physical activity

Mental activity

Methylated xanthines
   caffeine
   theophylline
   theobromine

Drugs
   antihypertensives
   tranquilizers
   sleeping pills
   hallucinogens

Social interaction

Suddenly, researchers began to put it all together in their search for aid to night-workers. Just as suddenly, researchers began to recognize that the information they discovered applied not only to shift-workers, but also to people suffering from jet lag, since the cause of *both* had their origins in a change in body clock rhythm and a massive disruption of sense of time, place, and well-being.

## CHAPTER FIVE

HOW THE THREE-STEP JET LAG PROGRAM WORKS

The program is called the Three-Step Jet Lag Program because it is divided into the three stages of your flight:

- Preflight
- Inflight
- Postflight

It combines all the knowledge scientists have gathered about rephasing body clocks ahead or backward through the combined use of the "major" external influences that are known to have a positive impact on the timing of body clocks: patterns of light and darkness, certain foods, periods of physical and mental activity, and methylated xanthines found in coffee or tea.

How does the program work? It begins with a **Preflight Step** of feasting and fasting (fasting meaning eating sparingly), starting from one to three days prior to take-off, depending on how much notice you have prior to your flight and how many time frames you will change; and it progresses into the **Inflight Step,** where you begin to reset your body's internal time clocks from the old time zone to the new time zone while on board the plane through the use of coffee and tea, periods of light and darkness, and periods of quiet and activity; and it concludes after you land with the **Postflight Step,** when you eat meals that are designed to see that you get the biggest boost of dependable energy possible during the day and the best possible sleep at night while you are in a new time zone.

It sounds simple because it is simple. The Three-Step Jet Lag Program will enable you to function optimally at home (while on the Preflight Steps), feel comfortable on the airplane (while on the Inflight Steps), and be able to enter into the mainstream of activity as soon as you land (while on the Postflight Steps), all with a minimum of effort.

Beating Jet Lag with Light

Whether you are fast asleep under a pile of blankets in a room with the shades down, or snug in a sleeping bag while camped out under the stars, when the electric light goes on, or the dawn breaks, you begin to enter the active phase of your twenty-four-hour daytime cycle. You have no choice.

As a daytime creature, like all other daytime animals on earth, you react when light strikes the eye; neurotransmitters are released that send an immediate signal to specific regions of the brain. In turn, these brain regions signal the rest of the body that your awake and active phase is about to begin.

Although man has tampered with the timing of the natural response to dawn and dusk through the development of darkened rooms and artificial light (which enable him to postpone rising for a few hours in the morning, and extend the amount of time he can be awake past sunset), he remains, genetically, a daytime animal exquisitely sensitive to light, and locked into its signals and timing.

The problem with rapid air travel is that when you undertake a long-distance flight that involves a time frame change, the wake/sleep cycle to which you have become habituated must shift accordingly. And it will, in due course. Old habits die hard, however. In the interim you will still want to fall asleep when your day would have ended back home and you will still want to rise when you normally would back home. It is a problem that has the potential to persist for days or weeks, disrupting your waking and sleeping patterns, making you fatigued when everyone else at your destination is wide-eyed, and keeping you awake when all the locals are retiring.

One of the keys, therefore, in the Three-Step Jet Lag Program is to use natural and artificial light to help resynchronize your wake/sleep schedule to the new time frame. With the Three-Step Jet Lag Program you do this in two of the three steps: while in the airplane and from the moment you arrive at your destination.

By pulling down the shade of a window seat while on board the plane during what would be nighttime at your destination—even if it is still daytime on your hometown schedule—and covering your eyes with an eyeshade or dark sunglasses to help shut out light from other windows or from people having the reading lights on, you can begin to **trick** your body into thinking it is in its new time zone already, and get the jump on reducing jet lag symptoms. Or, by turning on the plane's artificial light over your seat during what would be daylight hours at your destination, you can **trick** your body clocks into thinking it is daytime.

Since light stimulates you to keep awake, if you land (or before you arrive) at a destination and it is daylight out, you don't revert to your old time frame and take to your bed. Sequestering yourself in a darkened hotel room will only negate the benefits of the Jet Lag Program by perpetuating your old schedule. Instead, you expose yourself to the light so that it can help your body reset its internal clock.

Your motto is to "live as the Romans live" from the moment you arrive at your destination. If you are outdoors, you flood your eyes with daylight. No sunglasses. If you are indoors during daytime, you keep the artificial lights on. By saturating yourself in light, your diurnal/daylight neurotransmitters and hormones will be signalled to begin their proper course through you and fatigue will lift.

If it is nighttime when you arrive, again, you assume the destination schedule and get to your room, turn off the lights and shut your eyes until dawn. Most important, social cues and other signals to your active, daytime cycle will have been avoided. Soon enough, sleep will take over.

Beating Jet Lag with Foods

One of the major problems associated with jet lag is fatigue coupled with insomnia. You become so tired that you cannot enjoy the local sights or function up to par during the daytime. Yet, despite exhaustion, you find it difficult to get a sound night's sleep. Now, with the Three-Step Jet Lag Program, there are a number of excellent steps you can take to help you fall asleep or to keep you energized. One of these methods involves the intentional selection of certain foods to induce sleep or produce wakefulness.

Like everyone else, your state of sleepiness or wakefulness results from chemical changes in your brain that help "rev" you up or "slow" you down over the course of twenty-four hours. During the daytime, a combination of natural chemicals (the amino acid tyrosine, dihydroxyphenylalanine [L-DOPA], dopamine, norepinephrine, and epinephrine) are produced by your body and stimulate what is known as the adrenalin (or catecholamine) pathways in the billions of cells within your brain and in all other organ systems in your body. The adrenalin pathways insure that you *will* be active during the active phase of your day.

At night, the adrenalin pathway tends to become less dominant, and instead, another series of chemical combinations (tryptophan and serotonin) take over and constitute the indoleamine pathway in the brain. The indoleamine pathway, in turn, begins a sleep-inducing process that makes you drowsy and, ultimately, puts you to sleep. (Both pathways, by the way, are the targets of action for a variety of drugs, including antihypertensives, psychotropics, sleeping pills, tranquilizers, analgesics, and anesthetics.)

Researchers have shown that a meal composed primarily of **high-protein** foods, such as fish, fowl, eggs, meat, dairy products, and beans, stimulates the adrenalin pathway and gives you up to five hours worth of long-lasting energy. In contrast, a meal consisting principally of **high-carbohydrate** foods, such as pasta, salad, fruit, and rich desserts, gives you a surge of energy for up to an hour, but then actually encourages you, by influencing the indoleamine pathway, to go to sleep.

Thus, if you arrive in Austria in the morning after a long flight from the United States through many time zones, and have a breakfast of sugar-coated cereal and a sugar-sweetened beverage (all very high in carbohydrates), within the hour you will become fatigued and want to lie down. However, if you eat a hearty breakfast of steak and eggs, or an omelet, lean sausage, cheese, and milk (all of which are very high in protein), you stimulate the awake pathway and your body's active cycle. Taking the high-protein meal one step further, if you also have a high-protein lunch that includes lean beef, quiche (cheese), or fish steaks and milk, and avoid carbohydrates, you will virtually guarantee an entire day of sustained energy. Then, if you eat a high-carbohydrate supper of pasta, vegetarian salad, bread, and a rich dessert (and avoid or minimize protein intake), you will help prepare yourself, on a biochemical level, for sleep.

All that is required is the ability to sort out a menu (just ask the waiter to translate, if necessary), or to do your own shopping with high-protein breakfasts and lunches and high-carbohydrate suppers in mind.

Does this technique involve a great deal of self-discipline? Not if you realize that you are not really being denied any food during a particular day, but are simply postponing some favorite foods. Eventually, during the course of a given day, you may have *any* food you wish.

(As is dramatically evident in this illustration, high-protein breakfast [eggs, lean meat or fish, dairy products] sustains blood sugar energy throughout the morning. A high-carbohydrate breakfast [bread, doughnuts, sugar] results in immediate energy but leads to a rapid and drastic decline in blood sugar within an hour of breakfast. The effect of a high-fat breakfast is intermediate.) (Adapted from Dr. Raymond Greene, **Human Hormones**. London, 1970, p. 232.)

EFFECT OF VARIOUS CLASSES
OF FOOD ON BLOOD-SUGAR LEVEL.

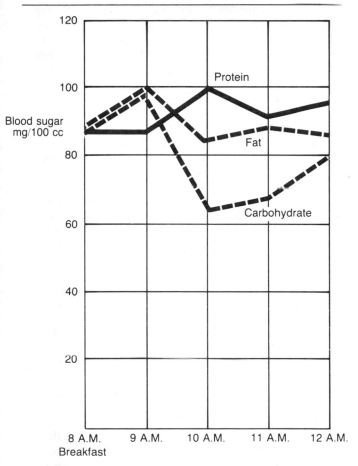

For the air traveler, high-protein breakfasts and lunches and high-carbohydrate dinners should be **de rigueur**, and anything else **verboten**.

Yes, you have to forego the "continental breakfast" (and you should keep that in mind when making hotel arrangements) of croissants or muffins slathered in jelly, or a typical "American" breakfast of grapefruit, sugar-coated cereal, sugar-sweetened orange drink and toast, or syrup-saturated pancakes or French toast—although you certainly can have any of these items toward evening. Eat greasy french fries,

61

mayonnaise, ketchup, and the like only sparingly during the day, but, again, feel free to indulge yourself at night in all those foods you denied yourself earlier. Have a huge pasta meal (no meat) at night; and as much wine and liquor as is sensible in the late afternoon and early evening. You will have more than enough energy, and then, as the evening winds down, you will wind down too.

Beating Jet Lag with Coffee or Tea

Using light and dark and special meals are but two aspects of the Jet Lag Program that minimize the effects of jet lag. Another very dramatic one is to use the chemical theophylline, which is found naturally in tea; and caffeine and theobromine, which are found commonly in coffee.

As amazing as it sounds, through their impact on the cellular time-keeping machinery, these three chemicals (which fall into the major category of "methylated xanthines") have an ability to reset body clock timers—to, in a sense, stop them cold and then push them ahead or backward.

On the basis of experiments with laboratory animals, scientists discovered a revolutionary fact: because your body changes biochemically over the course of a twenty-four- to twenty-five-hour day (the blond to red-head syndrome as described previously), you have different reactions to the same chemicals hour by hour. When methylated xanthines were administered to the laboratory animals in active phase (human "morning"), as if they had had a cup of black coffee, their body clocks' timing returned to that of an earlier time of day. The animals' average temperature dropped, and body functions slowed to levels characteristic of nighttime hours. If the methylated xanthines were given in mid-afternoon, there was very little effect on body clocks. When the methylated xanthines were given toward the evening hours, once again there was a dramatic reaction, only this time the body clocks' timing altered to that of a much later hour.

What did this discovery (revolutionary, by the way, for its time) mean to the jet traveler? Since the problem with jet lag revolves around body clocks having to speed forward (phase advance) or to turn back (phase delay) to adjust to destination time, scientists suspected that if a method could be developed to help rephase the body clocks rapidly either ahead or backward, the method would be a tremendous boon to the air traveler.

The natural chemicals found in coffee and tea now play a role in the Three-Step Jet Lag Program. For those people who can tolerate these natural chemicals, they offer another way to dramatically reduced jet lag symptoms. It is through their ability to affect simultaneously the billions of cells in each of the major organ systems of the body that these chemicals can help to rapidly resynchronize the hometown body clock to another time zone and enable you to cut days and weeks off jet lag.

There is only one slight hitch with the use of these chemicals. In order for methylated xanthines to be most effective, you have to give them up for a short time prior to taking them again, and program their use carefully. Depending upon how many time zones you are crossing, at certain times you will have to regulate your consumption of coffee, tea, cola, foods, or drugs containing methylated xanthines for one to three days. You will also have to initiate a special, but easy, feast/fast* pattern of eating to set the stage for the moment the Jet Lag Program calls for you to reintroduce methylated xanthines into your system.

While this part of the Program requires a certain amount of will power, it is a crucial part of it. Throughout the Program, the high-protein breakfasts and lunches, and high-carbohydrate suppers that you will eat will help insure energy throughout the day and a restful sleep at night, and theophylline, caffeine or theobromine (the methylated xanthines) will reduce the major trauma to your body clocks that time frame shifts produce.

The keys to the use of methylated xanthines are in the preparation of your energy reserves of glycogen in muscles and liver and in timing. They are to be taken in what is called a "punctuate," or quick and timely, fashion. The time of day you take them will vary according to the direction in which you are traveling and the number of time zones you will have changed by the time you get to your destination.

Products Containing Methylated Xanthines

While most people think coffee is the major source of caffeine, it is also found in large quantities in soft drinks, tea, and other products. Since you will have to avoid caffeinated products occasionally on the Jet Lag Program, the main caffeine-containing products (other than soft drinks) are listed below.

*"Fast," here, means "eating sparingly."

CAFFEINE CONTENT OF SUBSTANCES

Product	Quantity	Caffeine (in milligrams)
Coffee		
decaffeinated	5 oz.	2
instant, regular	5 oz.	53
percolated	5 oz.	110
drip	5 oz.	146
Tea		
one-minute brew	5 oz.	9–33
three-minute brew	5 oz.	20–46
five-minute brew	5 oz.	20–50
canned iced tea	12 oz.	22–36
Cocoa and chocolate		
milk chocolate	1 oz.	6
cocoa beverage (water mix)	6 oz.	10
baking chocolate	1 oz.	35
Non-Prescription Drugs		
stimulants		
Caffedrine capsules	standard dose	200
NoDoz tablets	standard dose	200
Vivarin	standard dose	200
pain relievers		
plain aspirin, any brand	standard dose	0
Anacin	standard dose	64
Midol	standard dose	65
Excedrin	standard dose	130
diuretics		
Pre-Mens Forte	standard dose	100
Aqua-Ban	standard dose	200
Permathene	standard dose	200
cold remedies		
Coryban-D	standard dose	30
Triaminicin	standard dose	30
Dristan	standard dose	32
weight-control aids		
Dietac	daily dose	200
Dexatrim	daily dose	200
Prolamine	daily dose	280

Source: *Consumer Reports*, October 1981, p.599.

Coffee. How much caffeine is in coffee depends on how it is brewed, how long it is brewed, and whether it is regular or instant coffee. As a rule, brewed coffee contains about twice as much caffeine as instant coffee. The drip method of brewing increases caffeine content over the percolator method.

Tea. The theophylline and caffeine content in tea depends on the type of tea leaves and the strength of the brew. If left to brew five minutes, for example, a cup of tea may have up to twice the caffeine equivalents of a cup that was brewed for one minute. As a rule, one cup of tea will have about one-fourth or one-third the caffeine equivalents of a cup of brewed coffee.

Chocolate. The cocoa bean contains natural theobromine. Theobromine content ranges from one to twenty milligrams per serving with an average content of ten milligrams per serving.

Over the Counter Drugs. Many drug products contain significant amounts of caffeine. Stimulants such as NoDoz and Vivarin are the equivalent of one or two cups of coffee. Pain relief, weight control, water-loss drugs can also contain large doses of caffeine.

Beating Jet Lag with Feasting and Fasting*

Two of the major keys in combating jet lag lie in the storage organs for energy reserves of the body, including the muscles and the liver, and the body's natural production of glycogen, which, in a very real sense, is the fuel of the human body. Experiments have shown that if glycogen reserves are allowed to run low through fasting or eating sparingly, you become highly sensitive to the ability of influences, such as light and darkness, food, and methylated xanthines, to shift the setting of your body clock rapidly to a new time frame.

Laboratory rats, for example, who were not fasted, but fed *ad libitum* (allowed to eat at will) and then exposed to a new lighting regimen that reflected an eight-hour time frame delay (as if they had undertaken a flight from Tokyo to Zaire, for example) took four to six days to resynchronize naturally. In contrast, in other laboratory rats, those not fed on the day before the time frame change, and then fed at the equivalent of breakfast time in Zaire, an extremely rapid shift to the new time frame occurred.

*"Fasting," here, means "eating lightly."

Combining this information with the discovery that methylated xanthines in coffee or tea had an ability to deplete the glycogen reserves in the liver even faster than simple fasting alone, scientists incorporated what they had learned about the impact of feasting and fasting, methylated xanthines, and the sudden appearance of food after a fast, into a comprehensive jet lag program.

Within the Jet Lag Program, you assume an on-again/ off-again pattern of feasting and fasting from one to three days prior to your trip, depending upon how many time frames you will change and how much advance notice you have of the flight. The Three-Step Jet Lag Program feast/ fast stage repeatedly replenishes the glycogen supply and then drains it, biochemically setting the stage for your body clocks to shift to a new time frame rapidly.

Beating Jet Lag with Physical and Mental Activity

In most living creatures, light is the fundamental time-setter and reinforcer of body clocks. One exception, however, is man. While light plays a powerful role in establishing or changing daily body rhythms, so do the effects of forced physical and mental activity. Having to get up and get out, whether to perform in the ballet or to catch a bus, actually cause chemical changes in the body that relate to stress and to the stimulation of unique neurotransmitters that help to keep you alert. Speaking to other people, socializing with them, "rubbing elbows," also precipitate the secretion of additional neurotransmitters that help body clocks resynchronize to a new time frame. Physically moving about, going to tour Versailles or the Kremlin, riding the Colorado rapids, or skiing the Alps, even if you are in a different time frame, will shake you out of lethargy and resynchronize your body clocks to the active phase.

With the Three-Step Jet Lag Program, the active phase is just that—active. If you are on the plane during what should be the active phase of the Three-Step Jet Lag Program, read, write, talk to your neighbor, stretch, move about. When you arrive at your destination, if your program calls for activity, even if you have the urge to slow down because your body clocks are in transition, keep walking and talking and you will help coerce your out-of-synchronization body clocks into speeding up the resynchronization process.

It works. Between 1975 and 1981, in a number of scientific papers from laboratories around the world, the Preflight, Inflight, and Postflight Steps involved in influencing body clocks were revealed, and the basis of the Three-Step Jet Lag Program was established. By incorporating the use of light and darkness, a specific composition of foods, periods of physical and mental activity, and methylated xanthines found in coffee or tea with a feast/fast regimen, scientists showed that multiple factors influencing body clocks could, indeed, have a dramatic impact on the severity and duration of jet lag-like symptoms.

It took over thirty years of research on an international and national level ultimately to amass all the disparate information and to organize it into the Three-Step Jet Lag Program, a system of relief that really works for the air traveler's most frequent complaint—jet lag.

In the pages that follow, the specific techniques you will use will be on the basis of the direction of your flight and the number of hours you will need to reset your watch, either ahead or back, when you arrive at your destination. It will not matter how many airplanes you have to take to get where you are going, or whether you take off late or spend hours circling the airport. The Three-Step Jet Lag Program will work, and work well, for everyone.

CHAPTER SIX

JET LAG
PROGRAM DIRECTIONS

The Three-Step Jet Lag Program consists of six jet lag programs to the east and six to the west. If your flight plan calls for an in-between time zone change, base your calculations on the next higher number.

Specifically, you have the following jet lag programs from which to choose. Remember, each time zone equals a one-hour difference in time.

Chapter Seven

Eastbound trips:	1–2 time zones crossed
Eastbound trips:	3–4 time zones crossed
Eastbound trips:	5–6 time zones crossed
Eastbound trips:	7–8 time zones crossed
Eastbound trips:	9–10 time zones crossed
Eastbound/westbound trips:	11–12 time zones crossed

Chapter Eight

Westbound trips:	1–2 time zones crossed
Westbound trips:	3–4 time zones crossed
Westbound trips:	5–6 time zones crossed
Westbound trips:	7–8 time zones crossed
Westbound trips:	9–10 time zones crossed
Westbound trips:	11–12 time zones crossed

(See **eastbound/westbound trips: 11–12 time zones crossed**, in Chapter Seven.)

Since each of these specific trips is subject to varying instructions within the Preflight, Inflight and Postflight Steps of the Three-Step Jet Lag Program, for every two time zones crossed, there is a detailed instruction sheet, as well as a Mercator map projection in which parallel spacing increases from the equator north and south, so that the shapes of coasts and small geographic features are closely preserved, and all compass directions from one place to another are correct throughout. This is the property that has made Mercator the standard navigation map from the time it was generally accepted (before 1600) up till now. On it a straight line represents constant compass directions. It shows the correct shapes of temperate zone regions, but exaggerates areas in polar regions.

Note also that there are some very exotic places highlighted on the maps as representative of potential trips. Although it is much more likely that your transmeridional travels will take you from London to Zurich, from Edinburgh to Frankfurt, from Paris to Athens, or perhaps even from Oklahoma City to Philadelphia more frequently than from Nome to Papeete or from Pago Pago to Santa Maria in the Azores, exotic destinations were included on the sample sheets for far more than purely romantic reasons. The places chosen represent the best aids that were available within their respective times zones that would provide a broad perspective of round-the-world travel.

NOTE: If you have no time to implement the Preflight Step of the Jet Lag Program, begin as soon as you can—preferably by the day of flight.

Questions to Ask Your Airline

Because you lose hours flying east or gain hours flying west, there are important questions to ask the airline representative when you call to book your flight:

1. What are your flight choices? Chapter Nine discusses the best departure time for your flights. Try to find an airline that will allow you the "ideal." However, you must also balance this choice against your arrival time.

2. What time will you be arriving? As will be explained later, arrival time is extremely important. Since the Jet Lag Program is designed to allow you to slip into the local time frame immediately upon arrival, if it is past your bedtime, destination time, you will have to be very active during a time when the program calls for sleep. Chapter Nine discusses the best time of arrival.

3. Will you have to set your wristwatch ahead or back? If ahead, you are flying in an easterly direction; if back, you are flying in a westerly direction.

4. How many hours are estimated for the entire flight? While not a crucial question, it is valuable to know the number of hours en route so that you can get a complete overview of your entire trip.

5. What time will meals be served and from what foods can you select? Airlines have a variety of meal options. Given notice, they can provide you with meals that are vegetarian, kosher, low-sodium, low-cholesterol, or high-protein. See what they offer so that you can begin to plan for high-protein breakfasts and lunches, and high-carbohydrate suppers.

Transfer the information given to you by the airline to the Itinerary Worksheet in Chapter Ten, or a photocopy of it. As soon as you have your itinerary laid out, mark your personal calendar accordingly, so that you can begin the Preflight Steps of the Jet Lag Program in plenty of time for full effectiveness.

Now you are ready to begin the specific instructions for your easterly or westerly flight. Plan ahead by familiarizing yourself with the overall approach—the feast/fast aspect—in particular, as well as when to and not to drink coffee or tea. Timing is important. Know ahead of time what's involved.

Know also that, as simple as the individualized plans (broken down into 2, 4, 6, 8, 10, 12 time zone changes, east and west) appear to be, by virtue of the fact that time itself becomes compressed or expanded, fractions of days enter the picture. For example, STEP TWO (morning of the flight) is not a clear cut day of twenty-four-hours because of the time changes going on as you fly across time zones. Therefore, STEP THREE (breakfast, destination time) can begin very quickly after step two, or can be delayed considerably. It all depends on how many time zones you cross and in what direction you are traveling.

Follow the directions of the individualized Three-Step Jet Lag Program for your particular flight. Remember, also, that Chapter Ten is devoted entirely to more complex flight plans, such as zig-zag flights, or multi-destination flights. No matter how complex the flight, OVERCOMING JET LAG should have an appropriate plan for you to follow. Jet lag is, indeed, a complaint relegated to the past.

## CHAPTER SEVEN

THE THREE-STEP JET LAG PROGRAM: EASTBOUND

EASTBOUND PHASE ADVANCE

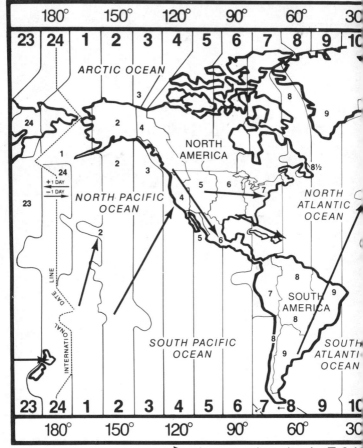

degrees longitude E & W

FROM:	TO:
Pago Pago [1]	Honolulu [2]
Papeete [2]	Los Angeles [4]
Vancouver [4]	Mexico City [6]
Denver [5]	Washington [7]
New Orleans [6]	San Juan [8]
Buenos Aires [9]	Santa Maria (AZ) [11]
Accra [12]	Frankfurt [13]
Rome [13]	Nairobi [15]
Manila [20]	Sydney [22]
Melbourne [22]	Wellington [24]

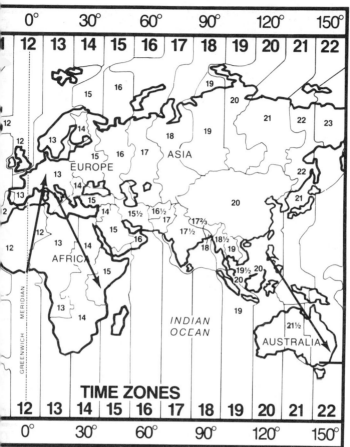

Greenwich Meridian

# TIME ZONES	mi/km	FLIGHT TIME (h)
1	2612/4204	4.5
2	4109/6613	7.1
2	2452/3946	4.3
2	1464/2356	2.5
2	1713/2757	3.0
2	6031/9707	10.4
1	3110/5006	5.4
2	3353/5396	5.8
2	3888/6258	6.7
2	1545/2566	4.5

Eastbound: One- to Two-Hour Time Zone Change

Although a one- to two-hour time zone change does not cause as much body clock upheaval as trips of a greater distance, even a one- to two-hour time zone change can produce jet lag symptoms that cause mild fatigue, poor appetite, gastrointestinal difficulties, and some confusion for a few days. To avoid jet lag symptoms completely, follow the simple steps outlined below. Also, don't forget to refer to the Composition of Foods table in Chapter Thirteen and the list of Major Influences on Body Clocks in Chapter Four.

FEAST = Generous servings
FAST = Limited portions

STEP ONE (preflight)

• TWO days before the flight, stop consuming beverages, food, or drugs containing methylated xanthines (coffee, tea, cocoa, chocolate, diet aids, etc.) in the early morning or late at night. If you want to have caffeinated beverages between three o'clock and four-thirty in the afternoon, feel free to do so.

• ONE day before the flight, eat a HIGH-PROTEIN breakfast, a HIGH-PROTEIN lunch, and a HIGH-CARBOHYDRATE supper. Because this is a fast day, keep the meals low in calories; a daily total of 800 calories is ideal.

• Shortly after six o'clock at night, DRINK TWO TO THREE cups of black coffee or strong, plain tea.

STEP TWO (morning of the flight)

• Get out of bed earlier than usual.

• SET A WATCH TO DESTINATION TIME and begin STEP THREE with breakfast, destination time.

STEP THREE (breakfast, destination time)

- A half-hour before breakfast, destination time, activate your body and mind (see Chapter Twelve, **Mental and Physical Exercise Program**). This is a feast day, so when you get up, eat a hearty, HIGH-PROTEIN breakfast, on destination time. Lunch should be a large, HIGH-PROTEIN meal, and supper a sizeable HIGH-CARBOHYDRATE meal.

- Drink water to compensate for the dehydration that is common on flights. Limit alcoholic beverages to no more than one drink (better yet, don't drink at all).

- Do not have any caffeinated beverages, foods, or drugs at all today.

- Since ten o'clock "old time" is midnight destination time, try and rest or sleep as soon as possible on destination time even if you do not feel tired. Wear a sleep mask if necessary.

EASTBOUND PHASE ADVANCE

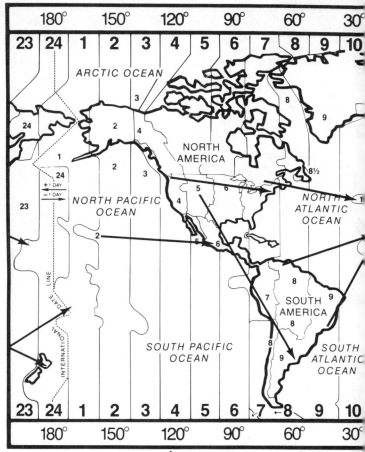

degrees longitude E & W

FROM:	TO:
Honolulu [2]	Mexico City [6]
Seattle [4]	Boston [7]
Denver [5]	Buenos Aires [9]
Montreal [7]	Santa Maria (AZ) [11]
Caracas [8]	Las Palmas [12]
Rio de Janeiro [9]	London [12]
Rome [13]	Delhi [17½]
Peking [20]	Wellington [24]
Tokyo [21]	Wake [24]
Sydney [22]	Pago Pago [1]

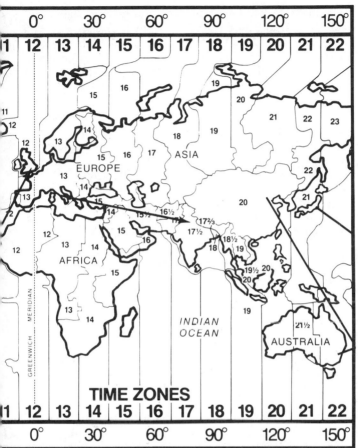

f Greenwich Meridian ↗

# TIME ZONES	mi/km	FLIGHT TIME (h)
4	3781/6084	6.6
3	2496/4016	4.3
4	5928/9538	10.3
4	2552/4106	4.4
4	3540/5696	6.1
3	5746/9248	9.9
4½	3685/5929	6.4
4	6698/10777	11.6
3	1983/3192	3.4
3	2733/4399	4.7

Eastbound: Three- to Four-Hour Time Zone Change

The three- to four-hour time zone change represents a significant jolt to your biochemical system. Even though you may consider a coast-to-coast United States flight or a continent-to-continent flight from Rio de Janeiro to London a minor trip, major jet lag symptoms are in store for you without the Jet Lag Program. Using the Three-Step Jet Lag Program for three- to four-hour shifts will greatly reduce the symptoms of jet lag. Since jet lag symptoms abate at different times and at different rates, by following the program outlined below, you will find that those symptoms that would have lingered a day or two may well be nonexistent and those symptoms that might have taken days or weeks to subside will end quite rapidly. Follow the simple steps outlined below. Also, don't forget to refer to the Composition of Foods table in Chapter Thirteen and the list of Major Influences on Body Clocks in Chapter Four.

FEAST = Generous servings
FAST = Limited portions

STEP ONE (preflight)

- THREE days before the flight, stop consuming beverages, foods, or drugs containing methylated xanthines (coffee, tea, cocoa, chocolate, diet aids, etc.) in the early morning or late at night. If you want to have caffeinated beverages between three o'clock and four-thirty in the afternoon, feel free to do so.

- The day before the flight, begin the feast/fast aspect of the Program, starting with the FEAST program of generous servings of a HIGH-PROTEIN breakfast and lunch, and a HIGH-CARBOHYDRATE supper.

STEP TWO (morning of the flight)

- Get out of bed earlier than usual.

- Eat a HIGH-PROTEIN breakfast, a HIGH-PROTEIN lunch, and a HIGH-CARBOHYDRATE supper. Because this is a FAST day, keep the meals low in calories; a daily total of 800 calories is ideal.

- Drink water to compensate for the dehydration that is common on flights. Limit alcoholic beverages to no more than one drink (better yet, don't drink at all).

- Shortly after six o'clock at night, no matter where you are or what you are doing, whether you are still in the airplane or not, DRINK TWO TO THREE CUPS of black coffee or strong, plain tea. Now RESET YOUR WATCH TO DESTINATION TIME.

- Since eight o'clock "old time" is midnight destination time try and rest or sleep as soon as possible—on destination time—even if you do not feel tired—until morning destination time. Put on a sleep mask if necessary.

STEP THREE (breakfast, destination time)

- Do NOT oversleep. A half-hour before breakfast, destination time, activate your body and brain (see Chapter Twelve, **Mental and Physical Exercise Program**).

- This is a FEAST day, so when you get up, eat a hearty, HIGH-PROTEIN breakfast on destination time. Lunch should be a large HIGH-PROTEIN meal, and supper should be a sizable HIGH-CARBOHYDRATE meal.

- Do NOT have any caffeinated beverages, foods, or drugs at all today.

- Keep active. Do NOT nap.

- Get to bed by ten-thirty in the evening, destination time.

- Under certain flight schedules, the reader may prefer for THIS day to be the flight day; if so simply shift each step of the above to one day earlier.

EASTBOUND PHASE ADVANCE

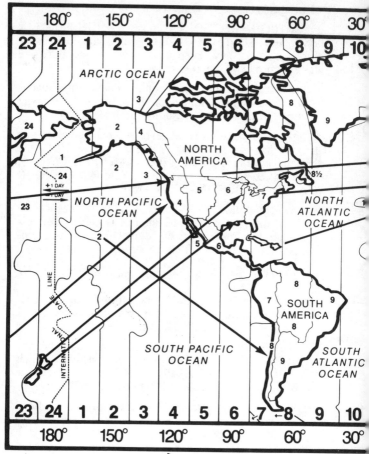

↖ degrees longitude E & W

FROM:	TO:
Honolulu [2]	Valparaiso [8]
Winnepeg [6]	Glasgow [12]
Boston [7]	Frankfurt [13]
San Juan [8]	Madrid [13]
Santa Maria (AZ) [11]	Calcutta [17½]
Cairo [14]	Singapore [20]
Tokyo [21]	Seattle [4]
Melbourne [22]	San Francisco [4]
Wellington [24]	New Orleans [6]
Auckland [24]	Chicago [6]

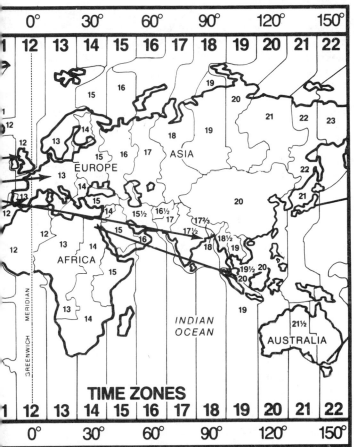

# TIME ZONES	mi/km	FLIGHT TIME (h)
6	6793/10930	11.7
6	3599/5791	6.2
6	3660/5889	6.3
5	3966/6382	6.9
6½	6549/10538	11.3
6	5088/8187	8.8
6	4790/7708	8.3
6	7854/12637	13.6
6	7794/12541	13.5
6	8309/13369	14.4

Eastbound: Five- to Six-Hour Time Zone Change

Anyone who has experienced the jet lag symptoms associated with a five- to six-hour time zone change knows they can become quite overwhelming. For this reason, travelers crossing the five-to-six time zones plus are usually the first to complain seriously about anticipated debilitation. They know that jet lag will be a significant problem with which they must reckon.

Again, you are bound to have symptoms, but with the Three-Step Jet Lag Program, they will be greatly minimized. Sleep, in particular, should be more easily obtained with the Jet Lag Program than without it. Follow the simple steps outlined below. Also, don't forget to refer to the Composition of Foods table in Chapter Thirteen and the list of Major Influences on Body Clocks in Chapter Four.

FEAST = Generous servings
FAST = Limited portions

STEP ONE (preflight)

- THREE days before the time change, begin the Program with a FEAST day by initiating HIGH-PROTEIN breakfasts, HIGH-PROTEIN lunches, and HIGH-CARBO-HYDRATE suppers.

- STOP consuming beverages, foods, or drugs containing methylated xanthines (coffee, tea, cocoa, or chocolate, etc.) in the early morning or late at night. If you want to have caffeinated beverages between three o'clock and four-thirty in the afternoon, feel free to do so.

- TWO days before the flight, eat a HIGH-PROTEIN breakfast, a HIGH-PROTEIN lunch, and a HIGH-CAR-BOHYDRATE supper. Because this is a FAST day, keep the meals low in calories; a daily total of 800 calories is ideal. Do NOT have any snacks after supper.

- The day before the flight, a FEAST day, allow yourself generous portions of foods based on the HIGH-PROTEIN breakfast and HIGH-PROTEIN lunch, and HIGH-CAR-BOHYDRATE supper plan. Do NOT have any snacks after supper.

STEP TWO (morning of the flight)

- Get out of bed earlier than usual.

- Eat a HIGH-PROTEIN breakfast, a HIGH-PROTEIN lunch, and a HIGH-CARBOHYDRATE supper. Because this is a FAST day, keep the meals low in calories; a daily total of 800 calories is ideal.

- Drink water to compensate for the dehydration that is common on flights. Limit alcoholic beverages to no more than one drink (better yet, don't drink at all).

- Shortly after six o'clock at night, no matter where you are or what you are doing, whether you are still in the airplane or not, DRINK TWO TO THREE CUPS of black coffee or strong, plain tea. Now RESET YOUR WRISTWATCH TO DESTINATION TIME.

- Since six o'clock "old time" is midnight destination time, try and rest or sleep as soon as possible on destination time—even if you do not feel tired—until morning destination time. Put on a sleep mask if necessary.

STEP THREE (breakfast, destination time)

- Do NOT oversleep.

- A half-hour before breakfast, destination time, activate your body and brain (see Chapter Twelve, **Mental and Physical Exercise Program**).

- This is a FEAST day, so when you eat, have a hearty HIGH-PROTEIN breakfast on destination time (remember: this meal usually occurs in flight). Lunch should be a large HIGH-PROTEIN meal, and supper should be a sizable HIGH-CARBOHYDRATE meal. Do NOT snack after dinner.

- Do NOT have any caffeinated beverages, foods, or drugs at all today.

- Keep active. Do NOT nap.

- Get to bed early, by ten o'clock at night, destination time.

EASTBOUND PHASE ADVANCE

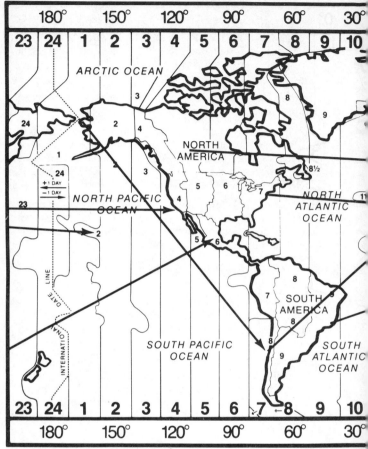

degrees longitude E & W

FROM:	TO:
Nome [1]	Valparaiso [8]
Edmonton [5]	Amsterdam [13]
New York [7]	Tel Aviv [14]
Valparaiso [8]	Moscow [15]
Rio de Janeiro [9]	Bombay [17½]
Reykjavik [12]	Shanghai ws[20]
Berlin [13]	Peking [20]
Calcutta [17½]	Honolulu [2]
Tokyo [21]	Los Angeles [4]
Melbourne [22]	Mexico City [6]

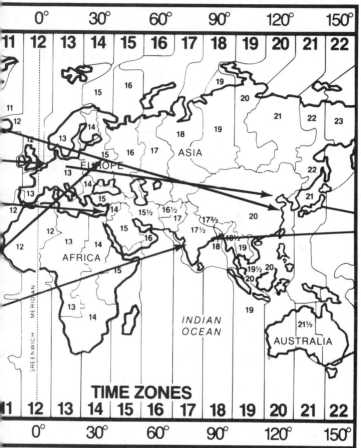

# TIME ZONES	mi/km	FLIGHT TIME (h)
7	8360/13451	14.4
8	4323/6955	7.5
7	5672/9126	9.8
8	8792/14146	15.2
8½	8257/13286	14.3
8	5559/8945	9.6
7	4567/7348	7.9
8½	5271/8481	9.1
7	5470/8802	9.5
8	8422/13551	14.6

Eastbound: Seven- to Eight-Hour Time Zone Change

A seven- or eight-hour time zone change causes severe jet lag symptoms that can virtually incapacitate you, mentally and physically, for days, if not weeks. On an easterly flight involving such a significant time change, you lose a large portion of sleep. For example, if you take an eight o'clock flight from Edmunton to Amsterdam, typically, you may be in the middle of a deep sleep (if you have not been up all those hours because of the excitement of the trip or the noise of the airplane) when it is time to land. When you land, after a greatly limited amount of sleep, it is time to function optimally to pass through customs, and time to get to your hotel or motel, etc. Getting up in the middle of the night and functioning coherently is not easy, but this is precisely what is called for in long-distance, multi-meridional flights. By following the simple steps outlined below, you should be able to step right into the mainstream of activity. Also, don't forget to refer to the Composition of Foods table in Chapter Thirteen and the list of Major Influences on Body Clocks in Chapter Four.

FEAST = Generous servings
FAST = Limited portions

STEP ONE (preflight)

- THREE days before the flight, begin the Program by initiating HIGH-PROTEIN breakfasts, HIGH-PROTEIN lunches, and HIGH-CARBOHYDRATE suppers.

- STOP consuming beverages, foods, or drugs containing methylated xanthines (coffee, tea, cocoa, or chocolate, etc.) in the early morning or late at night. If you want to have caffeinated beverages between three o'clock and four-thirty in the afternoon, feel free to do so.

- TWO days before the flight, eat a HIGH-PROTEIN breakfast, a HIGH-PROTEIN lunch, and a HIGH-CARBOHYDRATE supper. Because this is a FAST day, keep the meals low in calories; a daily total of 800 calories is ideal. Do NOT have any snacks after dinner.

- The day before the flight, a FEAST day, allow yourself generous portions of foods based on the HIGH-PROTEIN breakfast and HIGH-PROTEIN lunch, and HIGH-CARBOHYDRATE supper plan. Do NOT have any snacks after supper.

STEP TWO (morning of the flight)

- Get out of bed earlier than usual. Eat a HIGH-PROTEIN breakfast, a HIGH-PROTEIN lunch, and a HIGH-CAR-BOHYDRATE supper (you may want to skip this meal as breakfast destination time comes so soon). Because this is a FAST day, keep the meals low in calories; a daily total of 800 calories is ideal.

- Drink water to compensate for the dehydration that is common on flights. Limit alcoholic beverages to no more than one drink (better yet, don't drink at all).

- Shortly after six at night, no matter where you are or what you are doing, whether you are still in the airplane or not, DRINK ONE TO TWO CUPS of black coffee or strong, plain tea. Now RESET YOUR WRIST-WATCH TO DESTINATION TIME.

- Since four o'clock "old time" is midnight destination time try and rest or sleep as soon as possible on destination time—even if you don't feel tired—until morning time. Put on a sleep mask if necessary.

STEP THREE (breakfast, destination time)

- Do NOT oversleep. A half-hour before breakfast, destination time, activate your body and brain. (See Chapter Twelve, **Mental and Physical Exercise.**)

- DRINK ONE TO TWO CUPS of black coffee or strong, plain tea between six and seven-thirty in the morning, destination time, at destination time breakfast.

- This is a FEAST day, so when you eat, have a hearty, HIGH-PROTEIN breakfast on destination time. Lunch should be a large HIGH-PROTEIN meal, and supper should be a sizable HIGH-CARBOHYDRATE meal. Do NOT snack after dinner.

- Do NOT have any methylated xanthines at all today after breakfast.

- Keep active. Do NOT nap.

- Get to bed by ten o'clock at night, destination time.

EASTBOUND PHASE ADVANCE

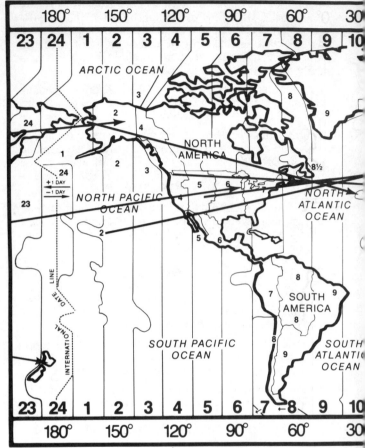

degrees longitude E & W

FROM:	TO:
Nome [1]	Santa Maria (AZ) [11]
Honolulu [2]	London [12]
Seattle [4]	Istanbul [14]
Denver [5]	Moscow [15]
Boston [7]	Sverdlovsk [17]
Santa Maria (AZ) [11]	Tokyo [21]
Reykjavik [12]	Melbourne [22]
Istanbul [14]	Wellington [24]
Volgograd [16]	Fairbanks [2]
Hong Kong [20]	Chicago [6]

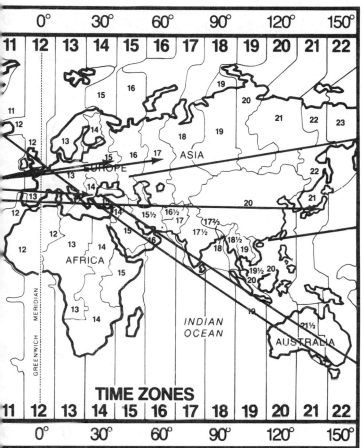

f Greenwich Meridian ⤴

# TIME ZONES	mi/km	FLIGHT TIME (h)
10	4954/7971	8.6
10	7226/11627	12.5
10	6061/9752	10.5
10	5485/8826	9.5
10	5025/8085	8.7
10	7247/11661	12.5
10	10544/16966	18.2
10	10663/17157	18.4
10	4560/7337	7.9
10	7790/12534	13.5

Eastbound: Nine- to Ten-Hour
Time Zone Change

The most significant problem associated with a huge time zone change such as a nine- to ten-hour time zone advance is the shattering of sleep and wake schedules. A nine- to ten-hour advance in time represents a switch from night into day or day into night. You are losing an entire night's sleep, and this holds true whether you are on the Jet Lag Program or not. Ten o'clock at night is eight o'clock in the morning, destination time! The problem, therefore, is how to handle not only the circadian phase change, but also the sleep deprivation, being awake for that entire time so that you can assume destination time activities right away. The key, of course, is to take advantage of the Three-Step Jet Lag Program. Follow the simple steps outlined below. Also, don't forget to refer to the Composition of Foods table in Chapter Thirteen and the list of Major Influences on Body Clocks in Chapter Four.

FEAST = Generous servings
FAST = Limited portions

STEP ONE (preflight)

- THREE days before the flight, begin the Program by initiating HIGH-PROTEIN breakfasts, HIGH-PROTEIN lunches, and HIGH-CARBOHYDRATE suppers.

- STOP consuming beverages, foods, or drugs containing methylated xanthines (coffee, tea, cocoa, or chocolate, etc.) in the early morning or late at night. If you want to have caffeinated beverages between three o'clock and four-thirty in the afternoon, feel free to do so.

- TWO days before the flight, eat a HIGH-PROTEIN breakfast, a HIGH-PROTEIN lunch, and a HIGH-CAR-BOHYDRATE supper. Because this is a FAST day, keep the meals low in calories; a daily total of 800 calories is ideal. Do NOT have any snacks after dinner.

- The day before the flight, a FEAST day, allow yourself generous portions of foods based on the HIGH-PROTEIN breakfast and HIGH-PROTEIN lunch, and HIGH-CAR-BOHYDRATE supper plan. Do NOT have any snacks after supper, and get to bed earlier than usual.

STEP TWO (morning of the flight)

- Get out of bed earlier than usual.

- Eat a HIGH-PROTEIN breakfast and a HIGH-PROTEIN lunch. Because this is a FAST day, keep the meals low in calories. You are only having two meals on the fast program, therefore a daily total of 400 calories is ideal. Do NOT eat again until destination time breakfast. Now RESET YOUR WRISTWATCH TO DESTINATION TIME.

- Drink water to compensate for the dehydration that is common on flights. Limit alcoholic beverages to no more than one drink (better yet, don't drink at all).

- Since two o'clock in the afternoon "old time" is midnight destination time try and rest or sleep as soon as possible on destination time—even if you don't feel tired—until morning destination time. Put on a sleep mask if necessary.

STEP THREE (breakfast, destination time)

- A half-hour before breakfast, destination time, activate your body and brain (see Chapter Twelve, **Mental and Physical Exercise Program**).

- Before breakfast (and no later than nine-thirty), DRINK TWO TO THREE CUPS of black coffee or strong, plain tea.

- This is a FEAST day, so when you eat, have a hearty, HIGH-PROTEIN breakfast on destination time. Lunch should be a large HIGH-PROTEIN meal, and supper should be a sizable HIGH-CARBOHYDRATE meal. Do NOT snack after supper.

- Keep active. Do NOT nap. Get to bed early.

EITHER WAY PHASE SHIFT

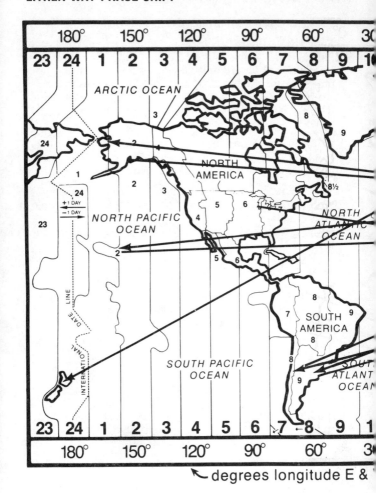

degrees longitude E &

FROM:	TO:
Honolulu [2]	Cairo [14]
Anchorage [2]	Amsterdam [13]
Chicago [6]	Calcutta [17½]
Valparaiso [8]	Peking [20]
Buenos Aires [9]	Singapore [20]
London [12]	Wellington [24]
Berlin [13]	Nome [1]
Istanbul [14]	Honolulu [2]
Manila [20]	Valparaiso [8]
Tokyo [21]	Buenos Aires [9]

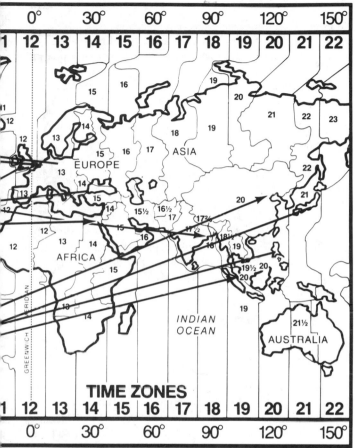

Greenwich Meridian ⌐↗

# TIME ZONES	mi/km	FLIGHT TIME (h)
12	8738/14060	15.1
11	4475/7201	7.8
11½	7981/12842	13.8
12	8088/13014	14.0
11	9864/15871	17.0
12	11682/18797	20.2
12	4342/6987	7.5
12	8104/13040	14.0
12	10930/17587	18.9
12	11400/18343	19.7

Eastbound and Westbound: Eleven- to Twelve-Hour Time Zone Change

In either direction, east or west, the eleven- to twelve-hour time zone change represents the most grueling body clock upheaval in transmeridional travel. Wherever your airplane lands in the world, when there has been an eleven- or twelve-hour time change, your body clocks must complete a 180-degree phase shift. When your body is programmed naturally to be asleep, it must now be forced to remain alert. When your body clocks normally see that you are bright-eyed and energetic, sleep must be induced. Indeed, all the mental and physical skills that peak and trough during the daytime and nighttime hours must now effect a total shift to a schedule that is not only new, but the complete opposite of the old schedule. Left to their own devices, in this instance body clocks can require literally weeks to reorganize and resynchronize. Not, however, with the Three-Step Jet Lag Program. Follow the simple steps outlined below. Also, don't forget to refer to the Composition of Foods table in Chapter Thirteen and the list of Major Influences on Body Clocks in Chapter Four.

FEAST = Generous servings
FAST = Limited portions

STEP ONE (preflight)

- THREE days before the flight, begin the Program by initiating HIGH-PROTEIN breakfasts, HIGH-PROTEIN lunches, and HIGH-CARBOHYDRATE suppers.

- STOP consuming beverages, foods, or drugs containing methylated xanthines (coffee, tea, cocoa, or chocolate, etc.) in the early morning and late at night. If you want to have caffeinated beverages between three o'clock and four-thirty in the afternoon, feel free to do so.

- TWO days before the flight, eat a HIGH-PROTEIN breakfast, a HIGH-PROTEIN lunch, and a HIGH-CAR-BOHYDRATE supper. Because this is a FAST day, keep the meals low in calories; a daily total of 800 calories is ideal. Do NOT have any snacks after supper.

- The day before the flight, a FEAST day, allow yourself generous portions of foods based on the HIGH-PROTEIN breakfast and HIGH-PROTEIN lunch, and HIGH-CAR-BOHYDRATE supper plan. Do NOT have any snacks after dinner. Drink caffeinated beverages only between seven and eleven-thirty in the morning this day.

STEP TWO (morning of the flight)

- Just before breakfast, and between seven and eleven-thirty in the morning, DRINK TWO TO THREE CUPS of black coffee or strong, plain tea.

- Eat a HIGH-PROTEIN breakfast and a HIGH-PROTEIN lunch (or skip lunch). Because this is a FAST day, keep the meals low in calories. You are only having one or two meals on the fast program, a daily total of 400 calories is ideal. Do NOT eat again until destination time breakfast. RESET YOUR WRISTWATCH TO DESTINATION TIME.

- Drink water to compensate for the dehydration that is common on flights. Limit alcoholic beverages to no more than one drink (better yet, don't drink at all).

- Since noon "old time" is midnight destination time try and rest or sleep as soon as possible—even if you do not feel tired—until morning destination time. Put on an eye mask if necessary.

STEP THREE (breakfast, destination time)

- A half-hour before breakfast, destination time, activate your body and brain. (See Chapter Twelve, **Mental and Physical Exercise Program**.)

- This is a FEAST day, so when you eat, have a hearty HIGH-PROTEIN breakfast on destination time. Lunch should be a large HIGH-PROTEIN meal, and supper should be a sizable HIGH-CARBOHYDRATE meal.

- Do NOT have any methylated xanthines at all today.

- Keep active. Do NOT nap.

- Get to bed by ten o'clock at night, destination time.

Questions and Answers

Q: Are you kidding? Drink two to three cups of black coffee or tea, and then go to sleep? How can I possibly do that after that much coffee or tea?
A: You probably won't fall sound asleep, and that's all right. The important thing is to relax. When you close your eyes and stop socializing, the chemical process that takes place in your body allows it to rest. Remember, the methylated xanthines are doing their job while you rest. Because of the methylated xanthines, when you enter the "active"

phase of the program, you will be well on your way to being synchronized with the new time frame. Quiet rest is just as effective as actual sleep.

Q: My usual approach to sleeping on the airplane is to drink a great deal of scotch. It works. I generally fall asleep. Why can't I keep drinking alcohol along with my coffee?
A: The information we have on the effect of alcohol on body clocks is somewhat inconclusive. Until more evidence is in, the best approach would be not to drink alcohol at all, or to drink very little while on the airplane. And don't forget, alcohol has a bigger kick because of the cabin's atmospheric pressures.

Q: On the fast days, must I eat everything offered, and as much as outlined?
A: No. The idea behind the fast days is to keep the caloric content down to a maximum of 800 calories. The high-protein breakfasts and lunches insure a high energy level throughout the day, despite the reduction in calories, and the high-carbohydrate suppers will actually help you sleep at night.

Q: I am watching my weight, and the "feast" days alarm me. Must I eat that much?
A: Yes. You don't have to eat everything suggested, but do eat enough to replenish your glycogen supplies, even if it is more than you usually eat. A few thousand calories is ideal, but that will depend greatly upon your own build and metabolism.

Q: I never eat breakfast. What should I do?
A: It is all right to miss breakfast on the fast days and the feast days, but be sure not to skip breakfast on the day of your arrival at your destination. You must eat a high-protein meal in order to signal your central nervous system that a new time frame has begun. If you do skip breakfast on preflight and inflight days and begin to feel a little weak, have an egg or a glass of milk (high in protein) to give you some energy.

Q: Why am I allowed to have coffee, tea, or caffeinated sodas between three o'clock and four-thirty in the afternoon, but not at any other time, unless specified by the Jet Lag Program?
A: Your body chemistry reacts differently to methylated xanthines over the course of a day. For reasons not yet fully understood, if taken in the morning, methylated xanthines have the ability to set body clocks back, and if taken at

night, ahead. If taken in the afternoon, "British tea-time," methylated xanthines seem to have little or no effect on the timing of body clocks.

Q: What about decaffeinated coffee and tea?
A: Have as much as you want at any time of the day or night. Since decaffeination removes the methylated xanthines, you don't have to worry about any effect on your body clock.

Q: What about sugar or sugar substitutes in my coffee or tea?
A: Sugar-free substitutes are fine. Just do not add real sugar or real cream to your coffee when the Program calls for three to five cups.

Q: What if I have to change flights, or get delayed. Does this throw the Program off?
A: Absolutely not. It does not matter if your flight is delayed in takeoff or landing, or if you have a layover. Just stick to the Program, and do the best you can.

Q: I really cannot tolerate coffee or tea in any amount whatsoever. Must I include them in the Program?
A: The methylated xanthines are extremely important to the Three-Step Jet Lag Program, but if you simply cannot tolerate even one cup of coffee, a half-cup of coffee, or a caffeinated diet soda, then skip it. At the hour you are supposed to have the beverage, don't have anything at all (of course, water is fine). Fast until breaking-the-fast at destination time.

Q: Would it help me sleep if I took a mild sedative after I drank my two to three cups of coffee? Is it a good idea to take a sleeping pill or tranquilizer on the night of my arrival at my destination?
A: Your body must work overtime to eliminate drugs from your system. You may think a sleeping pill or tranquilizer is helping you rest, but in reality you are introducing a factor that would confuse the orderly resetting of your body clocks.

Q: Maybe I should take a nonprescription stimulant on the day of my arrival. Will that help?
A: Many nonprescription stimulants have a caffeine base. Their use will confuse your body clocks, and you will negate the "clock-setting" effect of the caffeine.

Q: Will it be difficult to get high-protein breakfasts and lunches, and high-carbohydrate suppers while on the airplane?

A: The airlines have a special service for passengers with special food requirements: low-sodium, vegetarian, kosher, etc. If a particular meal that is served is not limited to strictly high-protein or high-carbohydrate foods, pick and choose among the foods offered. At lunch, for example, you may need to reject the roll, but certainly not the entire meal. Of course, you can always "brown bag" it.

Q: Why can't I take a nap on the first day at my destination if I feel a little tired?

A: The idea is to get right into the time frame of your destination. Studies have shown that a nap is, indeed, refreshing, although no one is quite sure why. (It is guessed that a break in conscious thought, an escape from anxiety or pressures, etc., may be the reason.) However, the nap disrupts sleep patterns later at night. Since you want to get a good night's sleep on your first night, avoid the impulse to nap.

Q: How soon after my flight has touched down may I drink caffeinated coffee or tea as often as I want?

A: You may drink them at any time between the hours of three o'clock and four-thirty in the afternoon, except during the days when they will be used to jolt your body clocks into a new time frame. On those days, consume coffee or tea only at the exact time they are called for in the Three-Step Jet Lag Program. Whether you resume old patterns of coffee or tea consumption after your day of arrival is up to you. However, the general consensus among scientists is that, since morning or evening consumption of methylated xanthines jolts body clocks ahead or back, by consistently drinking coffee or tea at these times of day, you put yourself in a perpetual state of circadian dyschronism—or disrupted body rhythms.

Q: What shall I do if my business meeting takes place in Germany, and then I have another business meeting a day or two later in Tokyo? How can I start a program for Frankfurt, get to Frankfurt, and then have to go on before I have had enough time to implement a new program for my next appointment?

A: Before you agree to these appointments, you should give the "timing" for the Jet Lag Program some serious thought. In this case, your options are (1) to reschedule enough time between appointments to enable you to implement the second program before you leave Germany, (2) to remain on Frankfurt time during your Tokyo appointment, or (3) to remain on your hometown time throughout the trip. Any course other than these three would have you at a distinct disadvantage in negotiation and decision-making abilities. Take a look at Chapter Ten, **Multi-Destination Flights.**

Q: I am on a restricted diet, and the foods recommended on the Three-Step Jet Lag Program are not always those my doctor insists on. What should I do?

A: The key to the food in the program is their composition and their timing. The program consists of high-protein breakfasts and high-protein lunches, followed by high-carbohydrate suppers. If you cannot follow the program exactly, then perhaps you can modify it, but keep to the high-protein, high-carbohydrate regimen for specific meals throughout the day. Consult with your doctor, and explain the mealtime approach. See what he or she says.

THE THREE-STEP JET LAG PROGRAM: WESTBOUND

WESTBOUND PHASE DELAY

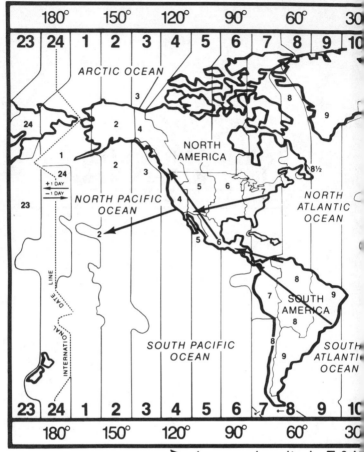

degrees longitude E & W

	FROM:		TO:
Los Angeles	4	Honolulu	2
Mexico City	6	Vancouver	4
New York	7	Phoenix	5
Rio de Janeiro	9	Panama	7
Caracas	8	Guatemala	6
Baghdad	15	Munich	13
Cairo	14	London	12
Teheran	16½	Moscow	15
Karachi	17	Addis Ababa	15
Sydney	22	Singapore	20

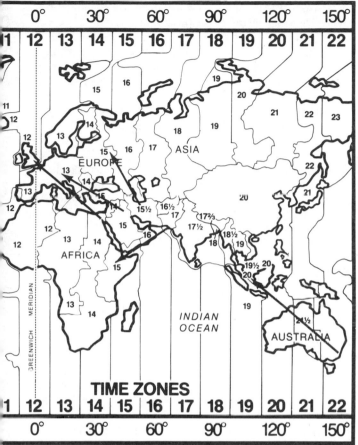

TIME ZONES

Greenwich Meridian ➚

# TIME ZONES	mi/km	FLIGHT TIME (h)
2	2551/4106	4.4
2	2448/3940	4.3
2	2029/3265	3.5
2	3289/5293	5.7
2	1609/2590	2.8
2	3170/1970	5.5
2	2192/3528	3.8
1½	1545/2486	2.7
2	2167/3486	3.4
2	3912/6296	6.8

Westbound: One- to Two-Hour Time Zone Change

For reasons that are not yet clearly understood by scientists and researchers, recovery periods after a westbound journey take significantly less time than recovery periods after an eastbound trip. It is suspected that you can adjust more readily to a schedule that expands the number of hours in a day than a schedule that condenses the number of hours in a day. When you fly in a westerly direction, you have the luxury of additional time to catch up on sleep. For example, when it is seven o'clock in the morning in Boston, when you encounter a time zone change in Chicago, you get to sleep until the equivalent of eight o'clock in the morning Boston time before you get up in Chicago. Nonetheless, any time zone change, even of an hour or two, produces symptoms you may wish to avoid. Follow the simple steps outlined below. Also, don't forget to refer to the Composition of Foods table in Chapter Thirteen and the list of Major Influences on Body Clocks in Chapter Four.

FEAST = Generous servings

FAST = Limited portions

STEP ONE (preflight)

- TWO days before the flight, stop consuming beverages, foods or drugs containing methylated xanthines (coffee, tea, cocoa, chocolate, diet aids, etc.) in the early morning or late at night. If you want to have caffeinated beverages between three o'clock and four-thirty in the afternoon, feel free to do so.

- ONE day before the flight, eat a HIGH-PROTEIN breakfast, a HIGH-PROTEIN lunch, and a HIGH-CARBO-HYDRATE supper. Because this is a fast day, keep the meals low in calories; a daily total of 800 calories is ideal. On this day caffeinated coffee or tea should be consumed between seven and eleven in the morning only.

STEP TWO (morning of the flight)

- On the day of the flight, immediately upon rising and up until 11 o'clock in the morning, begin drinking TWO TO THREE cups of black coffee or strong, plain tea. Do NOT have any more methylated xanthines today. Do NOT eat yet.

- SET A WATCH TO DESTINATION TIME and begin STEP THREE with breakfast, destination time.

STEP THREE (breakfast, destination time)

- A half-hour before breakfast, destination time, activate your body and mind (see Chapter Twelve, **Mental and Physical Exercise Program**).

- This is a feast day so eat a hearty HIGH-PROTEIN breakfast on destination time. Lunch should be a large, HIGH-PROTEIN meal, and supper should be a sizable HIGH-CARBOHYDRATE meal. Light snacks after supper are permissible.

- Drink water to compensate for the dehydration that is common on flights. Limit alcoholic beverages to no more than one drink (better yet, don't drink at all).

- Since midnight "old time" is ten o'clock in the evening destination time, try and rest or sleep as soon as possible on destination time. Wear an eye mask if necessary.

WESTBOUND PHASE DELAY

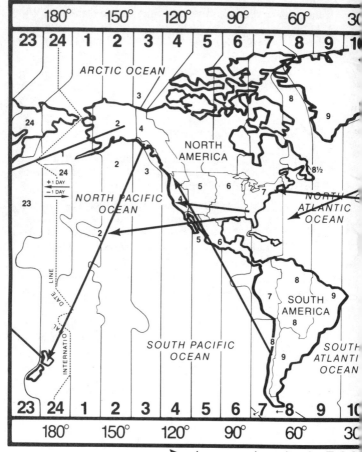

degrees longitude E & W

FROM:	TO:
Fairbanks [2]	Vladivostok [22]
Juneau [4]	Wellington [24]
New Orleans [6]	Honolulu [2]
Atlanta [7]	San Francisco [4]
Valparaiso [8]	Seattle [4]
Santa Maria (AZ) [11]	Boston [7]
London [12]*	Bermuda [8]
Teheran [16½]	Munich [13]
Colombo [17½]	Paris [13]
Wellington [24]	Hong Kong [20]

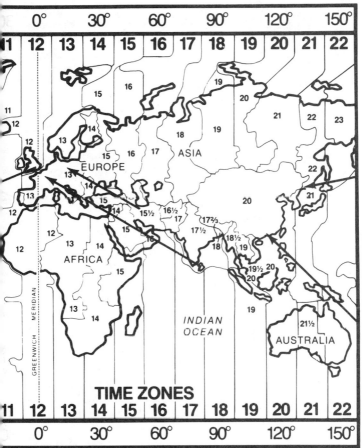

f Greenwich Meridian ⬏

# TIME ZONES	mi/km	FLIGHT TIME (h)
4	3305/5318	5.7
4	7475/12028	12.9
4	4207/6769	7.3
3	2139/3442	3.7
4	6230/10024	10.8
4	2436/3920	4.2
4	3428/5514	5.9
3½	2179/3507	3.8
4½	5292/8516	9.2
4	5853/9418	10.1

Westbound: Three- to Four-Hour Time Zone Change

Even though a three- to four-hour time zone change may still sound relatively insignificant, the body rhythm disruption it causes can be quite noticeable. For example, although it may only be subtle, for four days following landing at your destination, psychomotor performance will be affected, reducing hand—and eye—coordination. Or for five days, bowel and urinary function will be off schedule, making you very uncomfortable. Of course, since the Jet Lag Program has the capability of forcing rapid resynchronization, these problems should be virtually nonexistent. Follow the simple steps outlined below. Also, don't forget to refer to the Composition of Foods table in Chapter Thirteen and the list of Major Influences on Body Clocks in Chapter Four.

FEAST = Generous servings
FAST = Limited portions

STEP ONE (preflight)

• THREE days before the flight, stop consuming beverages, food, or drugs containing methylated xanthines (coffee, tea, cocoa, chocolate, diet aids, etc.) in the early morning or late at night. If you want to have caffeinated beverages between three o'clock and four-thirty in the afternoon, feel free to do so.

• ONE day before the flight, eat a HIGH-PROTEIN breakfast, eat a HIGH-PROTEIN lunch, and a HIGH-CARBOHYDRATE supper. Because this is a fast day, keep the meals low in calories; a daily total of 800 calories is ideal. On this day caffeinated coffee or tea should be consumed between seven and eleven o'clock in the morning only.

STEP TWO (morning of the flight)

• On the day of the flight, DRINK TWO TO THREE cups of black coffee or strong, plain tea no later than eleven-thirty in the morning. DO NOT have any more methylated xanthines today.

• SET A WATCH TO DESTINATION TIME and begin STEP THREE with breakfast, destination time.

STEP THREE (breakfast, destination time)

- A half-hour before breakfast destination time, activate your body and mind (see Chapter Twelve, **Mental and Physical Exercise Program**).

- This is a feast day, so eat a hearty, HIGH-PROTEIN breakfast on destination time. Lunch should be a large HIGH-PROTEIN meal and supper should be a sizable HIGH-CARBOHYDRATE meal. Light snacks after supper are permissable.

- Drink water to compensate for the dehydration that is common on flights. Limit alcoholic beverages to no more than one drink (better yet, don't drink at all).

- Since midnight "old time" is eight o'clock destination time, try and rest or sleep as soon as possible on destination time. Wear a sleep mask if necessary.

WESTBOUND PHASE DELAY

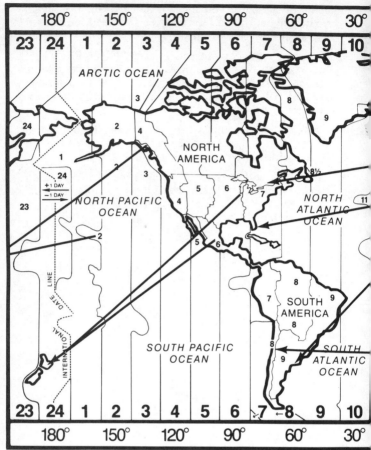

↖ degrees longitude E & W

FROM:	TO:
Honolulu [2]	Singapore [20]
Juneau [4]	Darwin [21½]
Mexico City [6]	Wellington [24]
Cape Town [14]	Valparaiso [8]
Copenhagen [13]	Montreal [7]
Moscow [15]	Buenos Aires [9]
Manila [20]	Istanbul [15]
Tokyo [21]	Moscow [15]
Chicago [6]	Wellington [24]
Madrid [13]	Miami [7]

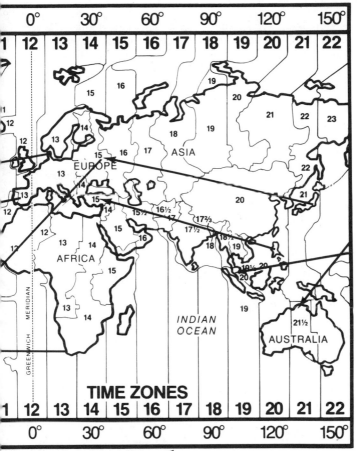

Greenwich Meridian ⤵

# TIME ZONES	mi/km	FLIGHT TIME (h)
6	6710/10797	11.6
6½	7105/11432	12.3
6	6899/11101	11.9
6	4998/8042	8.6
6	3604/5799	6.2
6	8375/13476	14.5
5	5659/9106	9.8
6	4657/7493	8.1
6	8349/13434	14.4
6	4417/7107	7.6

Westbound: Five- to Six-Hour Time Zone Change

By anybody's definition, a five- to six-hour time change represents a major upheaval in body clocks. Your entire biochemistry will have to shift by a quarter of the twenty-four-hour day. Sleep, waking, and eating schedules will all have to change to work with the new demands that will be placed on your body functions. Pay careful attention to the plan outlined below, however, and you will find your jet lag symptoms dramatically lessened, if not eliminated. Also, don't forget to refer to the Composition of Foods table in Chapter Thirteen and the list of Major Influences on Body Clocks in Chapter Four.

FEAST = Generous servings
FAST = Limited portions

STEP ONE (preflight)

- THREE days before the flight, begin the Program by initiating HIGH-PROTEIN breakfasts, HIGH-PROTEIN lunches, and HIGH-CARBOHYDRATE suppers. Since this is a FEAST day, allow yourself generous servings.

- STOP consuming beverages, foods, or drugs containing methylated xanthines (coffee, tea, cocoa, chocolate, diet aids, etc.) early in the morning or late at night. If you want to have caffeinated beverages, feel free to do so between three o'clock and four-thirty in the afternoon ONLY.

- TWO days before the flight, eat a HIGH-PROTEIN breakfast, a HIGH-PROTEIN lunch, and a HIGH-CAR-BOHYDRATE supper. Because this is a FAST day, keep the meals low in calories; a daily total of 800 calories is ideal. Do NOT have any snacks after supper.

- The day before the flight, a FEAST day, allow yourself generous portions of foods based on the HIGH-PROTEIN breakfast and HIGH-PROTEIN lunch, and HIGH-CAR-BOHYDRATE supper plan. Light snacks after supper are permissible.

STEP TWO (morning of the flight)

- On the day of the flight, sleep as late as possible. Immediately upon rising, DRINK TWO TO THREE CUPS of black coffee or strong, plain tea (no later than eleven o'clock in the morning). Do NOT have any more methylated xanthines today.

- Eat a "late" HIGH-PROTEIN breakfast, a "late" HIGH-PROTEIN lunch, and a "late" HIGH-CARBOHYDRATE supper. Because this is a FAST day, keep the meals low in calories; a daily total of 800 calories is ideal. Do NOT eat any snacks after supper.

- Drink water to compensate for the dehydration that is common on flights. Limit alcoholic beverages to no more than one drink (better yet, don't drink at all).

- RESET YOUR WRISTWATCH TO DESTINATION TIME.

- Since midnight "old time" is six o'clock in the evening destination time, prepare for a long day. Try and rest or sleep on destination time only.

STEP THREE (breakfast, destination time)

- A half-hour before breakfast, destination time, activate your body and your brain (see Chapter Twelve, **Mental and Physical Exercise Program**).

- This is a FEAST day, so when you eat have a hearty, HIGH-PROTEIN breakfast on destination time. Lunch should be a large HIGH-PROTEIN meal, and supper should be a sizable HIGH-CARBOHYDRATE meal. Light snacks after supper are permissible.

- Do NOT have any methylated xanthines today.

- Turn in at a reasonable hour, destination time.

WESTBOUND PHASE DELAY

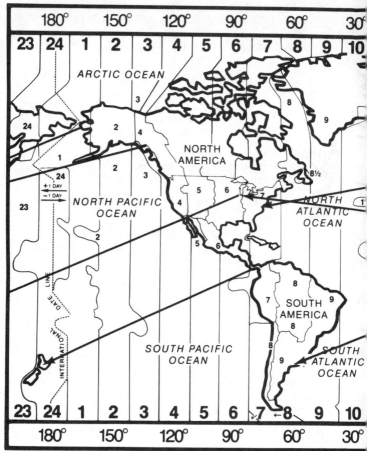

↖ degrees longitude E & W

FROM:	TO:
Nome [1]	Bombay [17½]
Juneau [4]	Hong Kong [20]
Chicago [6]	Darwin [21½]
Panama [7]	Wellington [24]
Cairo [14]	Chicago [6]
Moscow [15]	Washington [7]
Calcutta [17½]	Buenos Aires [9]
Hong Kong [20]	Berlin [13]
Tokyo [21]	Cape Town [14]
Melbourne [22]	Istanbul [15]

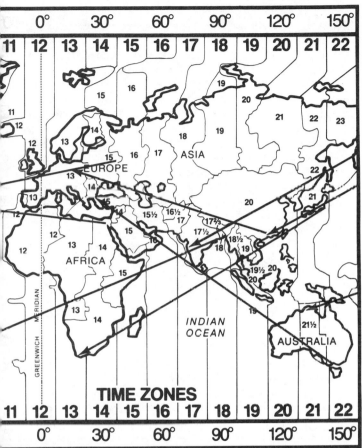

of Greenwich Meridian ↗

# TIME ZONE	mi/km	FLIGHT TIME (h)
7½	5901/9495	10.2
8	5634/9065	9.7
8½	9346/15038	16.1
7	7433/11960	12.8
8	6103/9820	10.9
8	4883/7857	8.4
8½	10242/16480	17.7
7	5500/8850	9.5
7	9071/14596	15.7
7	9088/14623	15.7

Westbound: Seven- to Eight-Hour Time Zone Change

A seven- to eight-hour time zone change westerly, like a seven- to eight-hour time zone change easterly, produces major body clock shifts in sleep and wake patterns. In order to assume destination time patterns immediately upon arrival, you should try to nap shortly after breakfast on the day of the time zone change because this time represents inactive periods at your destination also. Be aware that you are facing a very long day, seven or eight hours longer than your normal day. If you do not follow the Jet Lag Program, and, instead, allow yourself to fall asleep at your usual time, you will suffer the consequences of severe jet lag. The Three-Step Jet Lag Program will make it possible (and painless) for you to assume your destination schedule immediately. Follow the simple steps outlined below. Also, don't forget to refer to the Composition of Foods table in Chapter Thirteen and the list of Major Influences on Body Clocks in Chapter Four.

FEAST = Generous servings
FAST = Limited portions

STEP ONE (preflight)

- THREE days before the flight, begin the Program by initiating HIGH-PROTEIN breakfasts, HIGH-PROTEIN lunches, and HIGH-CARBOHYDRATE suppers. Since this is a FEAST day, allow yourself generous servings.

- STOP consuming beverages, foods, or drugs containing methylated xanthines (coffee, tea, cocoa, chocolate, diet aids, etc.) during the early morning or late evening. If you want to have caffeinated beverages, feel free to do so between three o'clock and four-thirty in the afternoon ONLY.

- TWO days before the flight, eat a HIGH-PROTEIN breakfast, a HIGH-PROTEIN lunch, and a HIGH-CARBOHYDRATE supper. Because this is a FAST day, keep the meals low in calories; a daily total of 800 calories is ideal. Do NOT have any snacks after supper.

- The day before the flight, a FEAST day, allow yourself generous portions of foods based on the HIGH-PROTEIN breakfast and HIGH-PROTEIN lunch, and HIGH-CARBOHYDRATE supper plan. Light snacks after supper are permissible.

STEP TWO (morning of the flight)

- On the day of the flight, sleep as late as possible. Immediately upon rising, and before eleven-thirty in the morning, DRINK TWO TO THREE CUPS of black coffee or strong, plain tea. Do NOT have any more methylated xanthines today.

- Eat a very "late" HIGH-PROTEIN breakfast. This is your first and last meal based your old schedule.

- Because breakfast is predicated on a FAST program, keep your breakfast meal low in calories; a total of 250 calories is ideal. Do NOT eat again until meal time on destination schedule, which, because of the time zone change, means you will be eating another breakfast based on destination time, only a few hours away because of your late breakfast. (Once you have your first breakfast, you will switch to the FEAST aspect of the Program in anticipation of breakfast, lunch, and supper on destination time.)

- Shortly after your late breakfast, rest, if possible, until your next meal, which is breakfast, destination time.

- Drink water to compensate for the dehydration that is common on flights. Limit alcoholic beverages to no more than one drink (better yet, don't drink at all).

- RESET YOUR WRISTWATCH TO DESTINATION TIME.

STEP THREE (breakfast, destination time)

- A half-hour before breakfast, destination time, activate your body and your brain (see Chapter Twelve, **Mental and Physical Exercise Program**).

- This is a FEAST day, so when you eat, have a hearty, HIGH-PROTEIN breakfast on destination time (remember: this meal usually occurs on the plane). Lunch should be a large HIGH-PROTEIN meal, and supper should be a sizable HIGH-CARBOHYDRATE meal. Light snacks after supper are permissible.

- Do NOT have any methylated xanthines today.

- Since midnight "old time" is four o'clock in the afternoon destination time, prepare for a very long day. Keep active. Do NOT nap. Try and rest or sleep on destination time only.

WESTBOUND PHASE DELAY

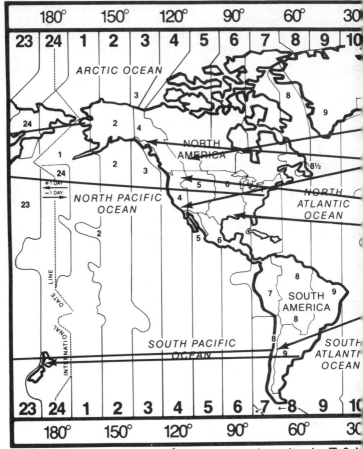

FROM: TO:

FROM:	TO:
Nome [1]	Moscow [15]
Tel Aviv [14]	Spokane [4]
Murmansk [15]	Edmonton [5]
New Orleans [6]	Manila [20]
Washington [7]	Vladivostok [22]
Valparaiso [8]	Melbourne [22]
Buenos Aires [9]	Wellington [24]
Warsaw [13]	Juneau [4]
Copenhagen [13]	Los Angeles [4]
Calcutta [17½]	Valparaiso [8]

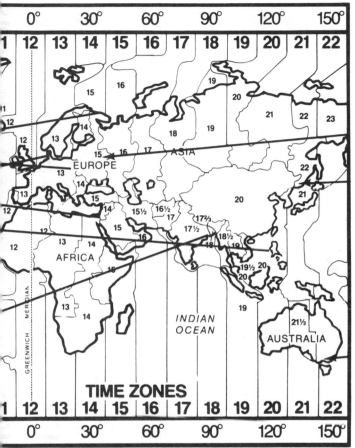

Greenwich Meridian ↴

# TIME ZONES	mi/km	FLIGHT TIME (h)
10	4036/6494	7.0
10	6685/10756	11.6
10	3800/61142	6.6
10	8724/14037	15.1
9	6485/10435	11.2
10	6998/11260	12.1
9	6260/10073	10.8
9	4680/7530	8.1
9	5612/9039	9.7
9½	10993/17688	19.0

Westbound: Nine- to Ten-Hour Time Zone Change

Like all the other larger time zone changes, the same problems exist, but simply become more severe. What you are going to be doing in this particular program is to try and grab as much rest during the flight day as possible, matching the inactive phase at your destination, and in anticipation of a very long day that entails being awake nine to ten hours longer than your normal schedule. You are going to need a great deal of energy to be up essentially for an entire day, but with the Three-Step Jet Lag Program, you should be able to fall into step with the local population quite easily. Follow the simple steps outlined below. Also, don't forget to refer to the Composition of Foods table in Chapter Thirteen and the list of Major Influences on Body Clocks in Chapter Four.

FEAST = Generous servings

FAST = Limited portions

STEP ONE (preflight)

* THREE days before the flight, begin the Program by initiating HIGH-PROTEIN breakfasts, HIGH-PROTEIN lunches, and HIGH-CARBOHYDRATE suppers. Since this is a FEAST day, allow yourself generous servings.

* STOP consuming beverages, foods, or drugs containing methylated xanthines (coffee, tea, cocoa, chocolate, diet aids, etc.) during the early morning or in the late evening. If you want to have caffeinated beverages, feel free to do so between three o'clock and four-thirty in the afternoon ONLY.

* TWO days before the flight, eat a HIGH-PROTEIN breakfast, a HIGH-PROTEIN lunch, and a HIGH-CARBOHYDRATE supper. Because this is a FAST day, keep the meals low in calories; a daily total of 800 calories is ideal. Do NOT have any snacks after supper.

* The day before the flight, a FEAST day, allow yourself generous portions of foods based on the HIGH-PROTEIN breakfast and HIGH-PROTEIN lunch, and HIGH-CARBOHYDRATE supper plan.

STEP TWO (morning of the flight)

- On the day of the flight, sleep as late as possible. Immediately upon rising, DRINK TWO TO THREE CUPS of black coffee or strong, plain tea. Do NOT have any more methylated xanthines today.

- Eat a HIGH-PROTEIN breakfast and a HIGH-PROTEIN lunch (or, better, skip lunch). Because breakfast and lunch are predicated on a "FAST" program, keep your meals low in calories; a total of 400 calories is ideal. Do NOT eat again until breakfast, destination time, only a few hours away because of the time change.

- Rest, if possible.

- Drink water to compensate for the dehydration that is common on flights. Limit alcoholic beverages to no more than one drink (better yet, don't drink at all).

- RESET YOUR WRISTWATCH TO DESTINATION TIME.

STEP THREE (breakfast, destination time)

- A half-hour before breakfast, destination time, activate your body and your brain (see Chapter Twelve, **Mental and Physical Exercise Program**).

- This is a FEAST day, so when you eat, have a hearty, HIGH-PROTEIN breakfast on destination time. Lunch should be a large HIGH-PROTEIN meal, and supper should be a sizable HIGH-CARBOHYDRATE meal. Light snacks after supper are permissible.

- Do NOT have any methylated xanthines today.

- Since midnight "old time" is two o'clock in the afternoon destination time, prepare for a very long day. Keep active. Do NOT nap. Try and rest or sleep on destination time only.

Westbound: Eleven- to Twelve-Hour Time Zone Change
(See Eastbound and Westbound Eleven- to Twelve-Hour Time Zone Change in Chapter Seven)

CHAPTER NINE

TIMING YOUR
DEPARTURE AND ARRIVAL

Which flight should you take to get from here to there? The answer involves the following three factors: the potential for sleep deprivation involved in getting up earlier than normal to catch a morning flight, or staying up later than usual to take an evening flight; the desire to have phase-shifted your body clock to destination time as soon as possible after your arrival; and how many flights are available from which to choose.

Avoid Sleep Deprivation. Sleep deprivation, no matter at which end of the day it occurs, begins to throw your body clocks off schedule and to precipitate the first stage of circadian dyschronism as your body clocks begin to go out of synchronization with one another. Ideally, you should pick a departure time that allows you to board the airplane at a reasonable hour in terms of your body clocks, neither forcing you to rise early nor keeping you up too late.

Ask About Arrival Time. As important as it is to not be sleep-deprived on the first day of your trip, it is also crucial to design an itinerary and flight plan that allow you to arrive at your destination during the "active" phase of the local residents, which, because of the Three-Step Jet Lag Program, will also be your active phase.

If you choose to arrive between midnight and dawn, destination time, then you will be forced to be very active immediately (disembarking, handling luggage, going through customs, taking ground transportation, checking in at a hotel, unpacking, etc.), at a time when you should be trying to sleep. All of this activity would be occurring at the very trough of the activity phase of the body clock cycle for all the local people, and since the goal of the Jet Lag Program is to synchronize you to local time frames immediately upon arriving, a nighttime arrival interferes with the synchronization process.

If a limited selection of flight plans requires that you arrive too late in the day for the "active" phase of the Jet Lag Program, and if you expect to conduct business in an intelligent manner, or enjoy yourself, at your destination, then it would be a better plan to depart one day earlier in order to provide time for a good night's sleep before conducting the next day's business.

Stated simply, the rule is to try to arrive sometime between eight o'clock in the morning and eight o'clock in the evening, preferably as close to eight o'clock in the morning as possible. Try never to arrive between midnight and five o'clock in the morning.

Preferred Departure Times
Keeping in mind the best times to arrive at your destination (see previous section), pick a flight tht departs as *early* as sensible when flying *east*, and as *late* as sensible when flying *west*. "Sensible" means within the normal home-time active phase of your circadian cycle.

Eastbound Arrival and Departure Times
For short trips east, don't lose too much sleep by getting up too early on the morning of the flight; for medium trips east, don't arrange a flight that forces you to awaken before five-thirty A.M.; and for long trips east, plan (a) a fairly late departure (though before midnight) and an arrival the next morning (anytime after six o'clock A.M., destination time), or (b) a very early departure (though after six A.M., home-time) and a very *late* arrival the same day (though before midnight, destination time).

Westbound Arrival and Departure Times
For short trips, be sure to sleep at least as late as usual, and preferably later. For medium trips west, you may sleep as late as the expected new rising time at your destination, and pick a compatible flight. For long trips west, arrange your departure so as to assure the longest possible interval of rest during the fast phase that precedes the en route high-protein breakfast that will coincide with breakfast time at your destination. If you can sleep well on board a transoceanic plane, or if a sleeper is available, then departure should be as early as possible (but after eight A.M.) to both reduce sleep deprivation during this very long day that accompanies flights west, and to provide for a prolonged interval of quiet and rest during the latter part of the fast that precedes destination time breakfast. Although a late departure before a long westbound trip allows you the luxury of a few additional hours of sleep early in the morning on the day of departure, thereby reducing the amount of sleep deprivation that you will accumulate, the late departure may deprive you of the rest you need during the late hours of your final fast period.

• • •

The Three-Step Jet Lag Program significantly shortens the duration of jet lag symptoms on the short haul, easterly/westerly flight of under six hours. However, as dramatically effective as the Program is, and even though it can greatly reduce the weeks it can often take to completely readjust to a new time frame, the Program does take a few days to do its job on extremely long flights involving multiple time zone changes.

That is why, if you are an athlete, or a concert performer, or even a diplomat who simply must be at his best at a specific time of day, you should plan to arrive at your destination early. How early? It depends upon how many time zones you have flown through, and whether you have traveled in an easterly or westerly direction, gaining or losing time.

What follows is a chart to help you plan your actual "day" of arrival, on the basis of your performance needs. Granted, everyone may not be able to afford the exact amount of time necessary for new body rhythms to become fully synchronized and locked into the new time frame, but every day, based on the chart, that you can allow yourself to recuperate and stabilize prior to your important appointment, will increase your mental and physical ability.

Best day of arrival

For Maximum Physical or Mental Performance After an Easterly Flight		
Time Zone Change	With Jet Lag Program	Without Jet Lag Program
+1	same day arrival	same day arrival
+2	same day arrival	same day arrival
+3	same day arrival	arrive one day early
+4	same day arrival	arrive two days early
+5	arrive one day early	arrive three to four days early
+6	arrive one day early	arrive four to six days early
+7	arrive two days early	arrive five to seven days early
+8	arrive two days early	arrive six to ten days early
+9	arrive two days early	arrive seven to eleven days early
+10	arrive three days early	arrive eight to twelve days early
+11	arrive three days early	arrive nine to twelve days early
+12	arrive three days early	arrive ten to twelve days early

For Maximum Physical or Mental Performance After a Westerly Flight		
Time Zone Change	With Jet Lag Program	Without Jet Lag Program
−1	same day arrival	same day arrival
−2	same day arrival	same day arrival
−3	same day arrival	arrive one day early
−4	same day arrival	arrive two days early
−5	arrive one day early	arrive three days early
−6	arrive one day early	arrive four days early
−7	arrive one day early	arrive five days early
−8	arrive one day early	arrive six days early
−9	arrive two days early	arrive seven days early
−10	arrive two days early	arrive eight to ten days early
−11	arrive two or three days early	arrive nine to eleven days early
−12	arrive three days early	arrive ten to twelve days early

CHAPTER TEN

MULTI-DESTINATION FLIGHTS

Whether you are zig-zagging across continents, or flying in a consistent direction around the globe, the Three-Step Jet Lag Program can be employed to great advantage. Although there are a number of variables that have to be taken into account, such as total overall length of the trip, number of days in any given location, whether it is a "round trip" journey, and the flexibility of your schedule once you arrive at your destination, with a little careful planning, you will be able to derive enormous benefit from the Program's techniques.

If you are going on a multi-destination flight, the first thing you should arrange is to have *two* wristwatches, or a companion who also wears a wristwatch. The next thing is to write down your itinerary, complete with approximate flying time, time changes involved in each flight, and the number of nights you will be spending in a specific destination. Here is an example:

Flights	Flying Time	Time Change	Nights at Destination
New York/Honolulu 1/30 10:50 A.M.– 5:00 P.M.	11 hours	+5	2 nights
Honolulu/Manila 12/2 1:50 A.M.– 7:25 A.M.	11 hours	+4	11 nights
Manila/Singapore 12/14 8:50 A.M.– 6:15 P.M.	9 hours	0	4 nights

After you write down all the itinerary details, you will have a better idea of the type of approach to take in combating jet lag with the Three-Step Jet Lag Program, and you will have a written reference for use during the actual trip.

The following are the types of choices you usually have. They are based on total number of days en route, and whether you are flying in a consistently easterly or westerly direction, or whether your journey takes you in a zig-zagging pattern, east to west and then west to east or vice versa.

Same direction
- Relatively brief length of stay
- Short stays

East/west direction
- Relatively brief length of stay
- Short stays

Any direction
- Long length of stay

Itinerary Worksheet

Flights	Flying Time	Time Change	Nights at Destination

Multi-Destination Flights, Same Direction—Short Stays

On short multi-destination flights in the same direction, you must decide whether you want to assume the time frame of your first destination or your second. You cannot do both; there simply is not enough time involved. For example, if you are traveling from Los Angeles to Hawaii for three days (time zone change −3) and then are going on to New Zealand for a total of three days (time zone change −2 from Hawaii), you could opt to synchronize your body clocks to Hawaii time, and stay on Hawaii time when in New Zealand, or you could plan to assume New Zealand time throughout the entire trip. It is up to you. Both methods work.

Flights	Flying Time	Time Change	Nights at Destination
Los Angeles/Hawaii		−3	3 nights
Hawaii/New Zealand		−2	3 nights
New Zealand/Los Angeles		+5	Returned

Again, do not forget to plan for a return trip to Los Angeles if you are going round trip. You must allow a sufficient number of days for the Preflight Steps of the Jet Lag Program.

Multi-Destination Flights, Same Direction— Relatively Brief Length of Stay

On a multi-destination flight, plan to adjust your body clocks to the destinations where you will stay the longest. For example, if you were flying from Chicago to India via Paris and Iran, and planned to spend only a few days in Paris, but a week or more in Iran, and then fly on to India for a day or two, your best bet would be to calculate the time zone changes from Chicago to Iran, and follow the Three-Step Jet Lag Program as if you were not stopping in Paris at all. You would shift to Iran time during the Chicago-to-Paris flight, and while in Paris, stay on Iran time. Just do your best to impose Iran time on your activities.

Flights	Flying Time	Time Change	Nights at Destination
Chicago/Paris		+7	2 nights
Paris/Iran		+2½	7 nights
Iran/India		+2	2 nights
India/Chicago		−11½	Returned

When you leave Iran for India, stay on Iran time while you are in India. Do not forget, if you plan to return from India, to select the appropriate Three-Step Jet Lag Program in sufficient time to use the Preflight Steps.

Multi-Destination Flights, East to West and West to East—Short Stay

Of course, the ideal approach is to allow sufficient time between time zone changes to prepare for each. However, in flights where you fly in a predominantly easterly or westerly direction, land for a brief one- or two-day visit, and then take to the air again, heading in the reverse direction, it is best to remain on home time throughout the trip. Taking off one day from Egypt, landing in Thailand (time zone change +5), turning around a few days later to embark for Spain (time zone change -3 from Egypt), only to return to Egypt a day or two later, creates a tremendously debilitating effect on body clocks if you try to synchronize them to a new destination, only to demand another resynchronization in another direction before the first attempt has been completed. A better approach would be to do your best to remain on hometown time throughout the trip, if at all possible. If conflicts arise (meetings, tours, etc.), at least try to keep within the hometown time frame as much as possible.

Flights	Flying Time	Time Change	Nights at Destination
Egypt/Thailand		+5	2 nights
Thailand/Spain		-7	2 nights
Spain/Egypt		+3	Returned

Multi-Destination Flights, East to West and West to East—Varying Lengths of Stay

There are a number of variables that have to be considered in multi-destination flights that zig-zag around the world and involve a varying number of days at each destination. Ideally, it would be best to think in terms of extreme time zone changes, amount of time involved in the Three-Step Jet Lag Program, and the number of days available at a destination for implementation. The following is an example of a flight that involves an east to west and west to east trip.

Flights	Flying Time	Time Change	Nights at Destination
New York/Honolulu		− 6	2 nights
Honolulu/Manila		− 6	11 nights
Manila/Singapore		0	4 nights
Singapore/Bali		0	5 nights
Bali/Hong Kong		0	4 nights
Hong Kong/Honolulu		+ 6	5 nights
Honolulu/San Francisco		+ 2	1 night
San Francisco/New York		+ 3	Returned

Notice that you have eleven days in Honolulu, followed by some insignificant time zone changes at your next few destinations, followed by another major shift as you fly back to Honolulu, but combined with five nights for adjustment, and with a final combined total of five time zone changes from Honolulu through San Francisco to New York.

The best way to handle this flight pattern is to stay psychologically and physiologically on New York time during the first two days in Honolulu, but begin the Three-Step Jet Lag Program Preflight Step in anticipation of commencing the Inflight Step while on the airplane to Manila. While in Singapore, Bali, and Hong Kong, just remain on local time, since it doesn't vary much from the time in Manila. Your eastbound flight from Hong Kong to Honolulu, however, involves another significant time zone change, so begin another set of Preflight Steps while still in Hong Kong, and implement the Inflight Steps while en route to Honolulu. Have a lovely, resynchronized five nights in Hawaii, and on the last few days of your stay, once again, start the Preflight Steps of the eastward-bound Jet Lag Program, breaking your fast on New York time, while still in San Francisco, and when you come down in New York, you should be ready to step right into the mainstream of activity with no problems.

Multi-Destination Flights, Any Direction—Long Length of Stay

A number of airlines offer fabulous flight-package arrangements. You buy a specific type of ticket that enables you to take as many flights as you desire, as long as you travel in essentially the same direction. Students, in particular, avail themselves of this type of flight package during the summer months, as do retired couples and world travelers with a great deal of leisure time. With the Three-Step Jet Lag Program, on trips that are going to require many weeks or months to complete, you will have the luxury of resynchronizing your body clocks to every destination upon arrival. When you have a few days before departure to begin the Preflight Steps, there is absolutely no reason to worry about wasting portions of your time with jet lag. On trips where scheduling is a little tight or virtually impossible, you must employ other measures that include superimposing one destination time on another. Not so, when you are traveling at your leisure.

Quite simply, write down your travel plans in the Itinerary Worksheet or fill it in as you go along. Start and stop the Three-Step Jet Lag Program as you plan to leave for a new destination and as you arrive. Just remember to allow sufficient time for the Preflight Steps.

## CHAPTER ELEVEN

AIR TRAVEL TIPS

Preflight

1. Check with airlines to see if they will supply you with high-protein breakfasts and lunches, and high-carbohydrate suppers for those meals you will be eating on hometown time while en route, and those meals consumed on destination time while en route.

2. Try to pre-select your seat in the airplane so that you are physically removed from the area of the galley, lavatories, and bassinettes (where lots of distracting activities and noises may interrupt your "rest" periods), try to arrange for plenty of leg room (near the emergency exits, in the front row of a section), and on the side of the plane opposite from where the sun will be when you are trying to sleep.

3. Pack the following items into a small bag to be carried onto the airplane: sleepshade, slipper socks, travel alarm, extra wristwatch (unless your normal wristwatch is of the type that can display two different time zones), toothbrush, toothpaste, razor, gum, lip balm, nasal decongestant, and **Overcoming Jet Lag.**

4. Pack a picnic basket of leftovers from the refrigerator in case meals served on the airplane do not correspond to the high-protein breakfast and lunch and high-carbohydrate supper program. Leftovers are also handy for light snacking inflight.

5. Wear loose clothing.

6. Do not let everything pile up until the last minute. Avoid tension, and get to the airport on schedule or with plenty of time to spare.

7. Try to avoid flying if you have a cold or ear problems. Remember that wine, sherry, or port contain histamines that can aggravate head congestion.

8. Check the weather at your destination and plan accordingly.

9. Consider using a small portable luggage cart as a "back-saving" device.

Inflight

10. Drink lots of fluids. The atmosphere in the airplane's cabin is literally as dry as the Gobi Desert.

11. If there are lots of empty seats on the airplane, make a quick move to a row of seats that can be converted into a quasi-bed for the "inactive" phase of the Jet Lag Program.

12. Reach for a pillow and blanket for the "inactive" phase of the Jet Lag Program. Covering yourself with a blanket helps keep you comfortable as your body temperature drops during inactivity. A pillow is a familiar psychological device that enhances your ability to sleep.

13. Loosen your clothing as an aid to circulation. Take off your shoes.

14. Avoid alcohol or limit it. Alcohol tends to add to the dehydration problem of poor cabin pressurization that pushes the humidity to as low as 5% or even 2%.

15. Eliminate or cut down on smoking. The carbon monoxide in cigarette smoke reduces the blood's ability to carry oxygen, and can cause headaches or slight dizziness while in flight.

16. If you wear contact lenses, consider removing them while in flight so that your eyes do not become irritated because of the extremely dry atmosphere in the cabin.

Postflight

17. Upon arrival, in your excitement at having landed at your destination, *do not* disregard the Postflight Steps of the Three-Step Jet Lag Program.

18. Remember to plan ahead for your next or return flight, and implement the Preflight Steps of the Jet Lag Program in plenty of time to assure the maximum benefits.

CHAPTER TWELVE

MENTAL AND PHYSICAL
EXERCISE PROGRAM

During some of the longer flights to a new time zone, the Jet Lag Program calls for periods of sleep or rest. At that time you should cease talking to your neighbor, close your book, or turn away from the inflight movie.

Once you have settled under a warm blanket and closed your eyes, your body will begin to slow down. Within a few minutes your heart rate will drop ten to twenty beats per minute. Without blood circulating vigorously throughout your body and brain, your temperature will begin to fall, your muscles and joints will stiffen and lose their elasticity, and your conscious mind will become sluggish. As you rest in your airplane seat, your legs, feet, and hands will swell slightly as gravity pulls the fluids in your body to your extremities.

After this rest period, the Jet Lag Program requires a few minutes of mental and physical exercise to bring your body and mind back to optimal functioning and alertness.

Waking Your Body in Time
For a New Time Zone

In order to follow the physical exercise aspect of the Jet Lag Program, you must *get up* and *get moving*. If you just remain seated in your chair, you will not be able to stimulate your heart so that your blood will begin to circulate rapidly, loosening up your joints and clearing your mind.

The following are a few physical exercises that can be done in the aisle, the rear of the plane, or in the lavatories. You should perform the exercises diligently in order to derive maximum benefits. (If you have back trouble or any physical ailment that will prevent you from exercising, check with your physician about participating in this aspect of the Program. Try to get substitute exercises.)

1. Take five deep breaths to pump your lungs full of oxygen and change the "tidal" air that is always in the bottom of your lungs.
2. Stand up on your toes and s-t-r-e-t-c-h for the ceiling. Repeat five to ten times.

3. Rotate your shoulders in both directions—left shoulder five times forward, five times backward; right shoulder five times forward, five times backward. Then rotate both shoulders simultaneously forward and backward.
4. Rotate your head—twice to the right, twice to the left. Repeat five times.
5. Bend backward from the waist, chin pointed toward the ceiling. Repeat five times.
6. Rotate your wrists and ankles. Repeat ten times.
7. Pull your knees up to your waist. Repeat five times for each leg.

Now, if you are not already thinking about a trip to the lavatory, or are not already there, go and tidy up, comb your hair, and splash cool water on your face. This step will also signal your body and mind that the day has, indeed, begun.

Waking Your Mind Up in Time
For a New Time Zone
Your blood is circulating, your muscles are stretched, and your joints are rotating smoothly. It is time to "flex" your mind and get it operating at peak performance.

1. If you are with friends or family or have made the acquaintance of seat companions or airplane personnel, dust off the mental cobwebs acquired during rest or sleep through stimulating conversation or a fast-moving game of cards that requires *concentration*.
2. If you do not want to talk with anyone sitting next to you (actually, if they are not participating in the Jet Lag Program, they may well be asleep and/or feeling the ill-effects of lack of rest or sleep), and you have an interesting book to read, do so. Or, if you have work to do, begin it. Work on something that requires concentration so that you do not drift back into a too relaxed state.

If you follow the advice in this chapter for mental and physical exercise, you will find that you are ready to begin a new day . . . on a new schedule . . . in a new time zone.

CHAPTER THIRTEEN

PUTTING YOUR OWN MENUS TOGETHER

On the Three-Step Jet Lag Program, food, in particular specific combinations of foods, plays a major role in eliminating chronic fatigue, ensuring limitless energy, and activating your body clock on the first day of arrival at your destination. While specific menus have been recommended with a variety of foods from which to choose (see pp. 149–151), the point may arise in your trip when you must concoct your own dishes or choose from a foreign menu.

The tables that follow are derived primarily from United States Department of Agriculture tables. They are a reliable guide to follow in formulating the HIGH-PROTEIN breakfasts and lunches and HIGH-CARBOHYDRATE suppers that are a crucial part of the Three-Step Jet Lag Program. Divided into columns representing caloric, protein, fat, and carbohydrate content, this section should provide you with all the information you need, whether at home or abroad, for developing your own Jet Lag Program menu.

If you are in doubt when consulting a foreign menu about the ingredients in a specific dish, ask the waiter to explain them to you. When the Program calls for high-protein meals, try to avoid rich sauces and condiments, which may well contain large amounts of oils and sugars, respectively.

When the program requires high-carbohydrate meals, realize that meat or cheese in any quantity has the power to change your body chemistry and promote energy—the last thing you want just prior to going to bed.

Yes, it takes a little investigation to determine the actual composition of meals, especially when a meal has many ingredients, but with a little perseverance and a little planning ahead of time, you should not have any trouble keeping your meals within the requirements of the Jet Lag Program.

COMPOSITION OF FOODS

	CALORIES	PROTEIN (grams)	FAT (grams)	CARBO-HYDRATES (grams)
MEATS AND POULTRY (3½ ounce servings)				
Bacon, crisp, drained:				
2 slices	86	5	8	1
Beef, cooked:				
Lean and fat	286	27	19	0
Lean only	196	31	7	0
Hamburger, broiled:				
Regular ground	286	24	20	0
Lean ground	219	27	12	0
Rib:				
Lean and fat	440	19	39	0
Lean only	241	28	13	0
Round:				
Lean and fat	261	28	15	0
Lean only	189	31	6	0
Steak, sirloin:				
Lean and fat	387	23	3	0
Lean only	207	32	8	0
Steak, porterhouse:				
Lean and fat	465	20	42	0
Lean only	224	30	11	0
Steak, T-bone:				
Lean and fat	473	20	43	0
Lean only	223	30	10	0
Steak, club:				
Lean and fat	454	21	41	0
Lean only	244	30	13	0
Beef, corned:				
Cooked, medium fat	372	23	30	0
Canned, lean	185	26	8	0
Beef liver, fried:	229	26	11	5
Cooked without fat	140	20	4	6
Beef tongue:				
Cooked, braised	244	22	17	trace
Canned or pickled	267	19	20	trace
Chicken, cooked:				
Broilers:				
Light meat, skinless	166	32	3	0
Dark meat, skinless	176	28	6	0
Roasters:				
Light meat, skinless	182	32	5	0
Dark meat, skinless	184	29	7	0
Canned, boneless	198	29	7	0
Livers, simmered	165	27	4	3
Lamb, choice grade:				
Leg:				
Lean and fat	279	25	19	0
Lean only	186	29	7	0
Loin:				
Lean and fat	359	22	29	0
Lean only	188	28	8	0

	CALORIES	PROTEIN (grams)	FAT (grams)	CARBO-HYDRATES (grams)
Shoulder:				
Lean and fat	338	22	27	0
Lean only	205	27	10	0
Pork, fresh; composite of trimmed, lean cuts:				
Medium fat class	373	23	31	0
Lean only	236	28	13	0
Chop, thick, with bone:	260	16	21	0
Roast, oven-cooked:				
Lean and fat	310	21	24	0
Lean only	175	20	10	0
Pork, cured:				
Ham, medium fat:				
Cooked, roasted	289	21	22	0
Lean only	187	25	9	0
Sausage:				
Bologna, all meat	277	13	23	4
Braunschweiger	319	15	27	2
Brown-and-serve	422	17	38	3
Country style	345	15	31	0
Deviled ham, canned	351	14	32	0
Frankfurters	304	12	27	2
Knockwurst	278	14	23	2
Liverwurst, smoked	319	15	27	2
Boiled ham, luncheon meat:	234	19	17	0
Polish-style sausage	304	16	26	1
Pork sausage, links	476	18	44	trace
Salami, dry	450	24	38	1
Sweetbreads:				
Beef	320	26	23	0
Calf	168	33	3	0
Lamb	175	28	6	0
Turkey:				
Flesh and skin, roasted	223	32	10	0
Light meat, skinless	176	33	4	0
Dark meat, skinless	203	30	8	0
Veal:				
Average cut, braised, lean and fat	235	28	13	0
Cutlet, boneless, broiled	185	23	9	4
Round, with rump	216	27	11	0
FISH AND SHELLFISH (3½ oz. servings)				
Abalone, canned	80	16	3	2
Anchovy, canned, 3 filets	21	3	1	trace
Bass, black sea, poached or broiled or baked without fat	93	19	1	0
Bass, striped, baked or stuffed	80	16	3	2
Bluefish, baked, broiled, fried	205	23	10	5

	CALORIES	PROTEIN (grams)	FAT (grams)	CARBO-HYDRATES (grams)
Clams:				
Raw, meat only	76	13	2	2
Canned, drained	98	16	3	2
Cod, broiled	170	29	5	0
Crab, Dungeness, rock, and king	93	17	2	trace
Flounder, baked	202	30	8	0
Haddock, fried	165	20	6	6
Halibut, broiled	171	25	7	0
Herring, raw:				
Atlantic	176	17	12	0
Pacific	98	18	3	0
Pickled	223	20	15	0
Salted or brined	218	19	15	0
Kippered	211	22	13	0
Lobster, northern, canned or cooked:	95	19	2	trace
Mackerel:				
Canned	183	20	11	0
Salted	305	19	25	0
Smoked	219	24	13	0
Mussels, meat only	95	14	2	4
Ocean perch, fried	227	19	13	7
Oysters, raw:				
Eastern	66	8	2	3
Western	91	11	2	6
Fried	239	9	14	19
Roe, baked or broiled, cod and shad	126	22	3	2
Salmon:				
Cooked, broiled or baked	182	27	7	0
Smoked	176	22	9	0
Scallops, bay and sea, steamed	112	23	1	0
Shad, baked	201	23	11	0
Shrimp, canned, meat only	116	24	1	1
Sole, baked	202	30	8	0
Swordfish, broiled	174	28	6	0
Tuna, canned:				
Packed in oil, drained	197	29	8	0
Packed in water	170	15	11	4
Weakfish, broiled	208	25	11	0
Whitefish, lake, smoked	155	21	7	0

FRUIT AND FRUIT PRODUCTS (½ cup except where otherwise noted)

	CALORIES	PROTEIN (grams)	FAT (grams)	CARBO-HYDRATES (grams)
Apples, 1 medium	70	trace	trace	18
Applesauce, fresh	60	trace	0	15
Applesauce, canned:				
Sweetened	91	trace	trace	24
k0 Unsweetened	41	trace	trace	11

	CALORIES	PROTEIN (grams)	FAT (grams)	CARBO-HYDRATES (grams)
Apricots:				
Canned, heavy syrup	86	trace	trace	22
Dried, uncooked	332	6	1	85
Cooked, sweetened, fruit and liquid	122	1	trace	31
Banana, 1 medium	85	1	trace	22
Blackberries, raw	58	1	1	13
Blueberries, raw	62	1	1	15
Cantaloupe, raw, ½ melon	40	1	trace	9
Cherries, raw, sweet	70	1	1	17
Cranberries				
Canned, sweetened	146	trace	trace	38
Juice, cocktail, canned	65	trace	trace	17
Figs, dried, 1 medium	60	1	trace	15
Grapefruit, raw, white,				
½ medium	41	trace	trace	11
Juice, fresh	41	1	trace	10
Canned, unsweetened	43	1	trace	10
Frozen concentrate, water added	44	1	trace	11
Grapes, seedless, green	69	1	1	16
Grape juice, bottled	66	trace	trace	17
Mandarin oranges, canned				
with syrup	50	1	trace	12
Nectarine, 1 medium	64	1	trace	17
Orange, 1 medium	60	2	trace	13
Orange juice:				
Fresh	45		trace	10
Frozen concentrate, water added	45	1	trace	11
Peaches:				
Fresh, 1 medium	33	1	trace	8
Canned, heavy syrup	96	trace	trace	25
Water packed	75	1	trace	19
Nectar, canned	48	trace	trace	12
Pears:				
Fresh, 1 medium	100	1	1	24
Canned, heavy syrup	76	trace	trace	20
Canned, water packed	32	trace	trace	12
Nectar, canned	52	trace	trace	13
Pineapple:				
Fresh, ½ cup	52	trace	trace	14
Canned, syrup	58	trace	trace	15
Canned, unsweetened	55	trace	trace	13
Plums:				
Fresh, 1 medium	30	trace	trace	7
Canned, syrup	83	trace	trace	22
Prunes:				
Dried, 4 medium	80	1	trace	19
Juice, canned	77	trace	trace	19
Raisins, dried	289	3	trace	77

	CALORIES	PROTEIN (grams)	FAT (grams)	CARBO-HYDRATES (grams)
Raspberries:				
Red, raw	57	1	1	14
Frozen, sweetened	98	1	trace	25
Strawberries:				
Fresh	37	1	1	8
Frozen, sweetened	109	1	trace	28
Tangerines:				
Fresh, 1 medium	46	1	trace	12
Juice, canned, unsweet-ened	43	1	trace	10
Frozen concentrate, water added	46	1	trace	11
Watermelon, 1 slim slice	26	1	trace	6
VEGETABLES (½ cup except where otherwise noted)				
Artichoke, cooked	44	3	trace	10
Asparagus, 6 spears	20	2	trace	3
Avocado, large, ½	180	2	17	6
Beans:				
Green, cooked	25	2	trace	6
Wax, cooked	22	2	trace	5
Lima, cooked	111	8	1	20
Red kidney, cooked	90	6	trace	16
Beets, cooked	32	1	trace	7
Broccoli, cooked	26	3	trace	5
Cabbage:				
Raw	25	1	trace	5
Cooked	20	1	trace	4
Carrots, diced, raw	42	1	1	10
Cauliflower, cooked	22	2	trace	4
Celery, diced, raw	17	1	trace	4
Corn:				
5″ ear	65	2	1	16
Cream style	82	2	trace	20
Canned, with liquid	66	2	1	16
Cucumber:				
Fresh, 1 medium	16	1	trace	3
Pickle, sweet, 1 medium	146	1	trace	37
Pickle, sour or dill, 1 large	11	1	trace	22
Eggplant, cooked	19	1	trace	4
Kale, cooked	39	5	1	6
Kohlrabi, cooked	24	2	trace	5
Lentils, cooked	106	8	trace	19
Lettuce, 2 large leaves	5	1	trace	trace
Mushrooms:				
Cooked or canned	17	2	trace	2
Raw	28	3	trace	4
Okra, cooked, 8 pods	29	2	trace	6
Olives:				
Green, 1 large	9	trace	1	trace
Ripe, 1 large	13	trace	2	trace
Onions:				
Mature, raw	38	2	trace	9
Cooked	29	1	trace	7

	CALORIES	PROTEIN (grams)	FAT (grams)	CARBO-HYDRATES (grams)
Parsnips, cooked	66	2	1	15
Peas, green:				
Cooked	71	5	trace	12
Canned, drained	88	5	trace	17
Frozen, cooked, drained	68	5	trace	12
Peppers, sweet, green,				
1 medium	22	1	trace	5
Potatoes, 1 medium				
Baked, skinless	90	3	trace	21
Boiled	105	3	trace	23
French fried, 10 pieces	155	2	7	20
Mashed, with milk	65	2	1	13
Chips, 10 pieces	110	1	7	10
Radishes, 4 small	10	trace	trace	2
Sauerkraut, canned	18	1	trace	2
Spinach, cooked	26	3	trace	4
Squash, cooked:				
Summer, diced	14	1	trace	3
Winter, baked	63	2	trace	15
Frozen, cooked, drained	63	2	trace	15
Sweet potatoes, 1 medium:				
Baked	155	2	1	36
Boiled	170	2	1	39
Candied	295	2	6	60
Tomatoes:				
Raw, sliced, 1 medium	22	1	trace	5
Canned or cooked,				
½ cup	22	1	trace	5
Juice, ½ cup	19	1	trace	4
Catsup, 1 tbsp.	15	trace	trace	4
Turnips, cooked, diced	23	1	trace	5
Vegetable juice, cocktail,				
6 oz.	31	2	trace	7
Vegetables, mixed, cooked,				
drained	64	3	trace	13

CHEESE, CREAM, MILK, EGGS, AND RELATED PRODUCTS

Cheese (1 ounce unless otherwise noted):				
American	106	6	9	1
Blue	100	6	8	1
Brie	95	6	8	trace
Camembert	85	6	7	trace
Cheddar	114	7	10	1
Cottage:				
Creamed, ½ cup	117	14	5	4
Uncreamed, ½ cup	96	20	1	2
Cream	99	2	10	1
Edam	101	7	8	1
Feta	75	4	6	1
Fontina	110	7	9	1
Gouda	101	7	8	1
Limburger	93	6	8	trace
Monterey jack	106	7	9	trace

	CALORIES	PROTEIN (grams)	FAT (grams)	CARBO-HYDRATES (grams)
Mozzarella	80	6	6	1
Muenster	104	7	9	1
Parmesan, grated, 1 tbsp.	111	10	8	1
Pot cheese:				
Low fat 2%, ½ cup	101	16	2	4
Low fat 1%, ½ cup	82	14	1	3
Port du Salut	100	7	8	trace
Ricotta, ½ cup	216	14	16	4
Romano	110	9	8	1
Roquefort	105	6	9	1
Swiss:				
Natural, domestic	107	8	8	4
Processed	95	7	7	1
Cheese spread, American	82	5	6	3
Cream, 1 tbsp.:				
Half-and-half	20	1	2	1
Light	29	1	3	1
Medium	37	1	4	1
Heavy	26	trace	3	trace
Sour	26	1	3	1
Creamer, nondairy, 1 tsp.	11	trace	1	1
Milk, fresh, 1 cup:				
Skim	72	7	trace	10
Skimmed partially, 2% fat	118	8	2	12
Whole, 3.7% fat	132	7	8	10
Yogurt, ½ cup:				
Plain, low fat	50	3	2	5
Whole milk	62	3	3	5
Eggs, chicken, 1 large boiled	79	6	6	1

GRAIN PRODUCTS: BREADS, CEREALS, GRAINS, CAKES

Biscuits, 1 medium	138	3	7	17
Bran flakes, ½ cup	303	10	2	81
Breads, 1 slice:				
Cracked wheat	60	2	1	12
French, enriched	58	2	1	11
Italian, enriched	55	2	trace	11
Protein	45	3	0	9
Pumpernickel, dark	56	2	trace	12
Raisin	60	2	1	12
Rye, light	55	2	trace	12
White, enriched	60	2	1	12
Whole wheat	55	2	1	11
Cakes, 1 medium slice:				
Angel food	110	3	trace	23
Apple Brown Betty	151	2	4	30
Chocolate fudge	420	5	14	70
Cupcake, plain	160	3	3	31
Fruitcake	105	2	4	17
Poundcake	130	2	7	16
Sponge	148	3	6	25
Cookies, plain, 1 medium	110	2	3	19

	CALORIES	PROTEIN (grams)	FAT (grams)	CARBO-HYDRATES (grams)
Cornbread	207	7	7	29
Cornflakes, enriched, 1 cup	93	2	trace	21
Corn muffins, 1 medium	155	4	5	22
Corn, puffed, presweetened, enriched, ½ cup	379	4	trace	90
Crackers, 2 medium:				
Graham	55	1	1	10
Saltines	35	1	1	6
Soda, plain	45	1	1	8
Donuts, plain, 1 medium	135	2	7	17
Macaroni, cooked, 1 cup	155	5	1	32
Melba toast, 1 slice	15	1	trace	3
Muffin, enriched, white flour, 1 medium	135	4	5	19
Noodles, cooked, 1 cup	200	7	2	37
Oatmeal, cooked, ½ cup	55	2	1	10
Pancakes, 1 medium	60	2	2	8
Pie, 1 medium slice				
Apple	330	3	13	53
Custard	265	7	11	34
Lemon meringue	300	4	12	45
Mince	340	3	9	62
Pumpkin	265	5	12	34
Popcorn, 1 cup	55	2	1	11
Rice, cooked, ½ cup:				
White, parboiled	100	4	trace	22
Puffed, enriched	25	trace	trace	6
Rice pudding, ½ cup	146	4	3	27
Rolls, 1 medium	115	3	2	20
Rye wafers, 2 medium	45	2	trace	10
Spaghetti, cooked, ½ cup	75	3	trace	16
Wheat, puffed, enriched, ½ cup:				
Plain, unsweetened	363	15	2	79
Presweetened	376	6	2	88
Wheat, shredded, plain, ½ cup	354	10	2	80
Wheat germ, 1 tbsp.	24	12	1	3
FATS, OILS, AND SHORTENINGS				
Butter, 1 pat	36	trace	4	trace
Margarine, 1 pat	36	trace	4	trace
Oils, salad or cooking, 1 tbsp.	125	0	14	0
Salad dressings, 1 tbsp.:				
Blue cheese	90	1	10	1
French	60	trace	6	2
Mayonnaise	110	trace	12	trace
Thousand Island	75	trace	8	1
MISCELLANEOUS ITEMS AND COMBINED INGREDIENTS				
Barbecue sauce, ½ cup	91	2	7	8
Beaver, cooked, 3½ oz.	248	29	14	0
Beef pot pie	246	10	15	19

147

	CALORIES	PROTEIN (grams)	FAT (grams)	CARBO-HYDRATES (grams)
Bouillon cube, 1	5	2	trace	trace
Candy, 1 ounce:				
Caramels	120	1	3	22
Chocolate, milk	145	2	9	16
Fudge	115	trace	3	23
Hard candy	110	0	0	28
Marshmallow	95	1	0	23
Chicken à la king	191	11	14	5
Chicken pot pie	235	10	14	18
Chili con carne, canned, beans, 1 serving	133	8	6	12
Chow mein, chicken, no noodles, 1 serving	102	12	4	4
Cole slaw, mayonnaise dressing, 1 serving	144	1	14	5
Fish sticks, frozen, cooked, 1 serving	176	17	9	7
Hollandaise sauce, 1 tbsp.	48	1	4	2
Ice cream, 1 serving	193	5	11	21
Lemonade, ½ cup	44	trace	trace	11
Lobster Newburg, 1 serving	194	19	11	5
Lobster salad, 1 serving	110	10	6	2
Macaroni and cheese, 1 serving	215	8	11	20
Nuts:				
Almonds, ½ cup	598	19	52	20
Brazil nuts, ½ cup	654	14	67	11
Cashew nuts, roasted, ½ cup	561	17	6	29
Coconut, dried, shredded, sweetened, 1 oz.	156	1	11	15
Peanuts:				
Roasted, salted, ½ cup	585	26	50	19
Peanut butter, 1 tbsp.	93	4	8	3
Pecans, chopped, 1 tbsp.	50	1	5	1
Walnuts, chopped, 1 tbsp.	50	1	5	1
Opossum, cooked, roasted, 1 serving	221	30	10	0
Pheasant, roasted, 1 serving	151	24	5	0
Pizza, 1 serving:				
Cheese topping	236	12	8	28
Sausage topping	234	8	9	30
Potato salad, 1 serving	145	3	9	13
Rabbit, stewed, 1 serving	216	30	10	0
Reindeer, hindquarter, 1 serving	256	19	19	0
Spaghetti, meatballs, tomato sauce, 1 serving	134	8	5	16
Sugar, 1 ounce	110	0	0	28
Tuna salad, 1 serving	170	15	11	4
Turkey pot pie	237	10	14	19
Waffles, mix, 2 medium size	356	9	2	76

Suggested Menus

Approximate Caloric Content = ( )

FAST Day

Breakfast:

1 egg, any style (82)
1/2 cup low-fat pot cheese or low-fat cottage cheese (86)
1/2 cup of orange juice (60)
Total calories: 228

or

2 eggs, any style (164)
1/2 piece of lightly buttered toast (50)
Total calories: 214

Lunch:

1/2 cup water-packed tuna or salmon with lemon juice (144)
1 piece of bread, lightly buttered or with a light coat of mayonnaise (65)
A few slices of tomato and a few leaves of lettuce (20)
1/4 cup low-fat or skim milk (75)
Total calories: 304

or

1 chicken breast, skin removed (154)
1 cup bouillon (5)
1/2 cup of low-fat pot cheese or cottage cheese (86)
Total calories: 245

Supper:

Medium-size plate of combination salad—lettuce, tomato, cucumber, onion, green pepper, radish, celery (120)
1 Tb. salad dressing, any kind (50)
1 piece of bread, lightly buttered (65)
1 alcoholic beverage (optional) (100)
1 apple or pear (50)
Total calories: 385

or

1 small bowl of pasta, lightly buttered with margarine (150)
1 piece of bread, lightly buttered (65)
1 cup cooked vegetables—string beans, summer squash, carrots, broccoli (40)
1 alcoholic beverage (optional) (100)
Total calories: 355

FEAST Day

(High caloric content important)

Breakfast:

Plenty of steak and eggs or ham and cheese
As much milk as you want
1/2 cup orange juice
1 piece of bread, lightly buttered

or

A large omelet, made with any ingredients—cheeses, vegetables
As much milk as you like
1 cup orange juice
1 piece of bread, lightly buttered

Lunch:

Lots of assorted cold cuts—chicken, turkey, lean meat, tongue
Assorted cheeses—any type and as much as you like
As much milk as you like
1 piece of bread, lightly buttered
1 cup vegetables—cauliflower, string beans, carrots
1 apple, pear, banana, bunch of grapes

or

Lots of meat, fish, fowl
Baked beans, lima beans
Slices of cheese, any kind, any amount
1 piece of bread, lightly buttered
1 apple, tangerine, cherries

Supper:

Pasta with a meatless tomato sauce, as much as you want
Bread, lightly buttered
Fruit salad, as much as you want of any fruit
Cake, cookies
Alcoholic beverages in reasonable amounts

or

Sauteed vegetables—potatoes, corn, green beans, onions, squash
Mixed salad—as much as you want
Salad dressing, any kind
Bread, lightly buttered
Cake, cookies
Alcoholic beverages in reasonable amounts

## CHAPTER FOURTEEN

SPECIAL PEOPLE/
SPECIAL INFORMATION

Shift-workers (Doctors, Nurses, Police, Fire Personnel, Factory Workers, etc.)

A "shift-worker," no matter what the shift, has a distinct advantage over other travelers when he or she opts to travel in an easterly or westerly direction. If you are already working the night shift, from midnight to eight A.M., for example, you are seven or eight hours "phase-advanced" from other travelers headed in the same direction. More than other travelers, you can step right into a new local time frame with little, if any, disruption of your body clocks or circadian rhythms.

The perfect example would be a trip from the United States to Europe. If you are a night shift-worker, your day begins about six or eight hours earlier than everyone else's in your community, and since a trip to London entails a time zone change of plus-six hours, you should be able to adjust to daytime life in England very, very easily.

If you are working the afternoon shift, from four P.M. to midnight, select a destination where your hometown nighttime is daytime someplace else, or about minus-eight time zones away in a westerly direction. Since you are already accustomed to being active at night, if you travel to a destination on nearly the other side of the world (the United States to Japan or Honolulu, for example), you should not experience any jet lag at all. All you really have to do is figure out where in the world the local daytime activities correspond to your normal active phase. It is easy.

Gamblers

Much of the gambling that takes place in casinos around the world begins in the evening hours and extends into the wee hours of the next day. Although many casinos are actually open twenty-four hours a day, the majority of the activity and the bigger crowds tend to descend upon the casino at night.

Whether you are an inveterate gambler or just an occasional dabbler, you would do well to consider your body clocks, along with your wallet or pocketbook, when you decide to take a seat at a gaming table. As a daytime creature disposed to perform best during daytime hours, if you are going to a casino where you will have to "turn night into day" by being up most of the night at your destination, pick a location where your body clocks can actually give you an advantage over other players. For example, if you are from New York, Philadelphia, or Miami, if you travel to Monaco or Evian (time change plus-six hours), when it is midnight at your destination, it is only six o'clock in the evening according to your body clocks. While everyone else at the tables is experiencing the onslaught of disrupted body clocks, you will still be wide-eyed and alert. If you are a West Coast resident and travel to Atlantic City in New Jersey, when it is two o'clock in the morning on the East Coast, and everyone is fading, it is only eleven o'clock in the evening, according to your body clocks.

In fact, it is far preferable to leave your hometown to gamble, even if your hometown is Las Vegas—where gambling takes place predominantly at night—and travel to another town where, again, you can have the advantages of the "active" phase of your daily rhythms during everyone else's "inactive" phase. The key would be to remain on hometown time throughout your gambling trip.

Athletes

The human body performs in cycles, performing certain tasks better at one time of the day than it does at another time of the day. For example, if you are going to perform a more mental task, such as balancing the checkbook, chronobiologists know that the best time to attempt it is between two and three o'clock in the afternoon. This is the proved period of increased mental acuity within the human's circadian or daily body rhythm. Therefore, if you are an athlete, in order to do your best, you have to know at what time of day you are going to be at peak physical prowess. The answer is throughout the active phase of the day, until about four or six o'clock in the afternoon. At any other time of day, you are working against your natural body rhythms, and you will not derive maximum benefits from exercise or practice.

When you are at home base, of course, you can tell what the best time is to perform or practice just by looking at the clock. If possible, you can schedule events with knowledge of circadian rhythms in mind, and know that you, indeed, are giving it your best shot. However, when you intend to compete after a rapid flight that involves a time frame change, you must allow your body rhythms to resynchronize to local time. If you do not, you will be competing with a body that simply cannot function optimally, and against competitors who are at a distinct physical advantage.

The Three-Step Jet Lag Program can and does force a rapid resynchronization, but realistically, the program cannot work an "overnight" miracle when severe time frame changes are involved. You must check the Best Day of Arrival chart in Chapter Nine and allow yourself (if it is at all possible) those few days required for the rapid resynchronization process to work. Arrive early enough at your destination to really get your body clocks well into synchronization *before* the event.

Also, a note about *burnout*. Sometimes athletes just seem to lose the ability to compete. When this is the case, poor sleep may be the culprit. Sleep loss can totally disrupt your timing, coordination, personality, and sense of well-being. The remedy for burnout may well be to go to bed, not back to the gym, when your athletic prowess seems to be waning. Regular sleep patterns are vital for maximum performance. Follow the Three-Step Jet Lag Program's high-protein breakfast and lunch, and high-carbohydrate supper plan. Almost overnight you should be able to stabilize your sleep/wake patterns.

Anyone Taking Drugs

Throughout the course of a twenty-four-hour day, levels of insulin, blood pressure, cholesterol, red blood cells, white blood cells, and other physiological properties and processes fluctuate. When a prescription label reads "take one in the morning" or "take one four times per day," the dosage is predicated on a scientific understanding of the human body's chemistry, and how it will react to the drug during a particular phase of your twenty-four-hour cycle.

New sleep/wake patterns, new meal times, and other conditions associated with time zone changes, result in discordance in your entire body chemistry. As your body chemistry changes, you become *more* or *less* sensitive to drugs, depending upon the state of your body chemistry. Occasionally, what was a beneficial dosage may even prove debilitating or fatal. **You must speak to your doctor about drug effects prior to flight.** If you are diabetic, hypertensive, or asthmatic, or if you are taking any drugs whatsoever for any reason, your medication dosage and timing must be adjusted to compensate for periods when internal body clocks are phasing forward or backward to synchronize to the new time frame.

Women

The menstrual cycle of women appears to be controlled by a number of environmental factors, including the light/dark patterns of the twenty-four-hour day. Many women who have irregular (or nonexistent) menstrual cycles are thought by chronobiologists to be out of synchronization with their environment. For example, flight attendants, doctors, nurses, fire and police personnel, and waiters, who work odd hours and in "shifts," often have to turn "night into day" and "day into night" in order to perform their jobs. Because humans are daytime creatures, working a night shift wreaks havoc with natural body rhythms, as does working a split-shift, or circumnavigating the globe.

For women with menstrual problems, the Three-Step Jet Lag Program may prove a boon because it literally forces the reestablishment of a defined daily body rhythm. The other side of the coin, however, is that a long-distance, rapid flight to a new time zone will disrupt a stabilized menstrual rhythm. But, in both cases, the Three-Step Jet Lag Program can remedy the situation.

The Elderly

As human beings get older, many circadian or daily rhythms alter or slow down measurably. Sleep, for example, tends to become fragmented, and the metabolic rate can decrease by as much as 30%. Although scientists are not exactly sure what the cause or causes may be, the theory is that the overall degenerative process inherent in aging also takes its toll on body rhythms, causing them to operate less efficiently and in poorer synchronization as the years go by. For this reason, shifting body clocks to a new time frame after a lengthy east or west flight may prove to be a very difficult ordeal for the elderly, particularly without the Jet Lag Program.

However, the Three-Step Jet Lag Program has the potential to help the elderly resynchronize their body clocks. For the first time in many years, perhaps many decades, the elderly should be able to assume a better-defined pattern of daily rhythms that results in a real feeling of improved well-being. All the ailments associated with disrupted daily body clocks (irritability, fatigue, constipation, headache, insomnia, inability to concentrate, etc.) should improve markedly, once body rhythms fall back into proper synchronization. The Three-Step Jet Lag Program could prove helpful indeed to the elderly.

Pilots and Air Crew Members

Some pilots and air crew members take to their beds immediately upon landing at their destination. They pull down the shades, turn off the lights, possibly take a drink or a sleeping pill—and hope for the best in sleep. Others never take a nap, but plunge right into destination time activities, and as the day proceeds, they proceed to enter a stage of exhaustion and circadian chaos. In other words, each crew member has his own remedy and methodology for dealing with jet lag. Some crew members give in to jet lag, and others fight it. But who fares best? The answer is neither.

Nor is the situation likely to change soon, at least not with the current flight options and rest periods that are available to flight personnel. The pilot or air crew member who has flown through the night is physically exhausted from being up all day and all night, and is now combining natural exhaustion with body rhythm dyschronism. When he gets to his hotel, the best he can hope for is a nap. There is no way his sleep will be anything but fragmented and inadequate. By taking a drink or a sleeping pill, in actuality, he exacerbates the problem. Drugs (and sleeping pills and alcohol are drugs) may make your eyes close and may make you lose consciousness, but the sleep they promote is woefully inadequate. In fact, drugs cause the body, whether in a state of consciousness or unconsciousness, to work hard to rid itself of alien chemicals during the time it should be totally involved in the recuperative sleep process. So you wake up as tired or more tired than before. Also, recent research has shown that there is a hangover effect associated with the commonly used sleep-inducers that lasts much longer than originally thought. Twenty-four hours after taking an over-the-counter sleep remedy, the effects can still be felt. The Jet Lag Program will be useful only when there is time for implementation: during a leave of absence, while on a vacation, or if a large block of time exists between flights.

However, there are a number of relaxation techniques available, which, in fact, do help promote relaxation and sleep. Of course, putting these techniques into effect requires some education, motivation, and self-discipline. The following is a list of techniques that pilots, crews, and cabin attendants have reported as useful.

Relaxation Response. Likened by some authorities to the techniques of transcendental meditation, the relaxation response was described by Herbert Benson, M.D., of the Harvard Medical School. Dr. Benson has you sit upright in a comfortable position (although some people prefer to lie down) close your eyes, and repeat the word "one" over and over again. Through this constant repetition, you eliminate extraneous thought from your consciousness, and begin to feel a sense of calm and well-being which often progresses to sleep. When you awake or arise, you feel refreshed. Since the relaxation response technique does not involve a change in lifestyle or philosophy, it is easy to implement.

Autogenic Training Technique. Developed by J. Schultz about sixty years ago and refined over the years by W. Luthe, the Autogenic Training Technique involves repeating suggestions of warmth and heaviness over and over again. This technique has been used in studies of insomniacs and does, indeed, prove to be very effective in reducing the amount of time it takes to fall asleep. It also seems to enhance the quality of that sleep. As a byproduct, it has been found that physiological and emotional tolerances are increased as well.

Hatha Yoga. Hatha yoga is considered the most basic type of yoga you can master. Concerned mainly with physical postures ("asanas"), hatha yoga involves assuming a variety of positions, either standing, sitting, or lying down (on your back or front), which enable you to relax through breathing exercises, and ultimately, to sleep. Not to be confused with other branches of yoga, for example Kundalina or Raja yoga, which involve the spiritual, more than the physical, hatha yoga works well as a relaxation technique with full benefits realized after postures are perfected.

Supersonic Travelers

In 1927, Charles Lindbergh flew a single-engine Ryan, "The Spirit of St. Louis," from New York across the Atlantic to Paris in a grueling 33 hours and 30 minutes at 116 miles per hour. In 1946, the DC4 accomplished the same trip in 23 hours and 45 minutes at 217 miles per hour. In 1957, the Super Starliner arrived in Paris in 14 hours and 40 minutes at 328 miles per hour. In 1959, the Boeing 707 completed the flight in 8 hours at 558 miles per hour. In 1977, the Concorde touched down in 3 hours and 45 minutes at 1,350 miles per hour.

During his visit in 1982 to Washington, D.C, for discussions with President Ronald Reagan about problems in Central America, French President François Mitterand crossed the Atlantic on an Air France Concorde at twice the speed of sound. Mitterand's visit was reported by the press to be "as quick and simple as flying across the Atlantic for lunch." By the clock, he had, in fact, arrived in the United States an hour before he left France. Of course, the effectiveness of this kind of "quicky visit" depends entirely upon the round-trip traveler conducting all his business during his own normal active daytime phase (happily coinciding, in this instance, with the active daytime phase of the people visited), and in returning home to his bedside before his own normal sleep-onset.

However, when you take the Concorde, and do not return home right away there are several Jet Lag Program options from which to choose. One is to remain in the United States for several days, on "Paris" time. For example, you would get up six hours earlier than everyone else in the eastern time zone, and go to bed six hours earlier each evening for the duration of the trip. Meals would be light and taken on Paris time. Exercise and social events would also have to be on Paris time. All late-night festivities and gala receptions would have to be avoided.

Another option is to initiate the Three-Step Jet Lag Program after arrival. For example, you can let the swift flight day on board the Concorde be the feast day and the next day be the fast day (still on Paris time), then break the fast with breakfast on destination time two days after arrival.

Similar options are open to the New York executive flying east by the Concorde to conduct business in Brussels on New York time. If he or she elects to stay longer in Europe, all that must be done is that the Three-Step Jet Lag Program should begin on any day that is convenient to the revised schedule.

Midnight Fliers

The Red-Eye Express—and all other variations of flight that require staying up very late to catch the flight—disrupts sleep patterns as significantly as the changing of time zones. It may be economical, but the midnight flight wreaks havoc with your body's natural rhythms and body clocks.

In order to counter the problems of the late-night departures, you should implement the Three-Step Jet Lag Program as you would for any daytime or early evening flight from coast to coast. When traveling in an easterly direction (California to New York), when the Program calls for "methylated xanthines," take them as scheduled, stay awake until you get on the airplane, and then rest or sleep as soundly as possible. The fact that your plane does not take off until very late at night, or the wee hours of the morning, should not interfere with the actual timing of the Program. When traveling in a westerly direction (New York to California), the morning of the flight drink the "methylated xanthines" as prescribed, and continue the Program accordingly, slipping onto California time with breakfast on destination time, and remaining alert until sleep time on the West Coast.

Travelers By Sea

It is anticipated that there will be one billion dollars worth of new tonnage, and a 50% growth in the number of passengers taking cruises over the next three years. If you have the time and the inclination, cruising may well be the most advantageous way to avoid jet lag on easterly and westerly journeys. When you cruise, if you leave by ship from your *own* time zone, you do not get severe jet lag symptoms. Ships move too slowly. By the time your ship drops anchor at its final destination, you will have naturally, over the course of your days at sea, become synchronized with the local time frame, and you will not need any jet lag program at all. However, if your cruise begins after a long transmeridional flight (Europe, Asia, Australia to the Caribbean, for example), make sure you implement the Three-Step Jet Lag Program that is appropriate for your point of departure by *ship*. If you are cruising and then flying, begin the Preflight Steps, in sufficient time, while on board the ship.